Richard B. Gunderman

Leadership in Healthcare

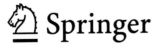 Springer

Richard B. Gunderman, BA, PHD, MD (Hons), MPH
Indiana University Medical Center
Indianapolis, IN
USA
rbgunder@iupui.edu

ISBN: 978-1-84800-942-4   e-ISBN: 978-1-84800-943-1
DOI 10.1007/978-1-84800-943-1

British Library Cataloguing in Publication Data
A catalogue record for this book is available from the British Library

Library of Congress Control Number: 2008937458

Printed on acid-free paper

Springer Science + Business Media
springer.com

Foreword

Leadership in Healthcare by Richard Gunderman is a marvelous and much needed book that examines the essential role of leadership in the future of the medical profession. As Gunderman notes in the first chapter: "To think outside the box, we need to read and converse outside the confines of our discipline." Dr. Gunderman is eminently well qualified for the challenge of thinking outside of his discipline. In addition to his M.D. from the University of Chicago, Dr. Gunderman also earned a Ph.D. in Social Thought from the University of Chicago. This combination of medical and philosophical training gives Dr. Gunderman a unique perspective from which to explore the field of Leadership in Healthcare. With his unusual preparation and wide-ranging intellect, Dr. Gunderman has already had a profound impact on many fields, including philanthropy, ethics, bioethics and medicine. With this book he will extend his influence into the field of leadership studies.

Dr. Gunderman's ability to weave together the insights from the fields of medicine and philosophy and add perspectives from literature and film makes this treatise essential reading not only for those interested in medical leadership but also for the broad area of leadership studies. In *Leadership in Healthcare* Dr. Gunderman draws from such disparate sources as Aristotle, William Harvey, Jane Austen, Andreas Vesalius, Søren Kierkegaard and Akira Kurosawa to craft a powerful argument on the role of leadership in the profession of medicine.

In his famous essay, the *Hedgehog and the Fox*, Isaiah Berlin suggested that all great thinkers could be divided into one of two camps: hedgehogs or foxes. The hedgehogs "know one big thing." They have a single integrating paradigm through which they view the entire world. They see the world through a single integrating lens. According to Berlin, thinkers such as Dante, Lucretius and Pascal were hedgehogs. On the other hand, foxes "know many things." They view reality from a multitude of different perspectives. Famous foxes include Herodotus, Shakespeare and Pushkin. As I read *Leadership in Healthcare*, I see Dr. Gunderman as a fox lamenting the fact that medicine has become dominated by hedgehogs.

This book is long overdue. An in-depth understanding of the role of Leadership in Healthcare is critical both for the field of medicine and for the larger society. As citizens of developed societies age and become wealthier, the role of medicine will inevitably become larger and more important. Healthcare currently consumes over 16% of the GDP of the United States and is projected to grow to at least 20% of the GDP within 10 years. At the same time medical training has become increasingly more specialized. Although specialization is vitally important, it is also crucial to have generalists, people who span the narrow and artificial boundaries and are concerned with the organic nature of the enterprise. If too few professionals are concerned about the "big picture" of their profession, it can enter into a death spiral in which specialization begets more specialization. The net result is that the overall health of the larger system can suffer and even fail.

Dr. Gunderman has a very insightful chapter on the role of organizations in the future of medicine. Organizational structures that may have been appropriate in earlier decades may be wholly inappropriate today and for the future. Just a few decades ago, the modern business corporation had literally dozens of layers of bureaucracy. Today, those organizations that have survived tend to be considerably flatter with far fewer layers of bureaucracy. At one time most of corporate power was concentrated in a single leader. Today power tends to be dispersed to multiple leaders. Some of the more successful organizations now include external stakeholders in decisions that, at one time, were purely internal. Overall, developed societies have seen a dramatic shift from authoritarian organizational systems to democratic systems.

The issue of appropriately aligning incentives and rewards for physicians can be generalized to many other professions. For example, there are those who argue that the 2008 economic downturn was in large part caused by the decoupling of the traditional relationships between bankers and home buyers. As recently as two decades ago, many home loans were originated by local banks who loaned to local homebuyers. The bankers had a very strong incentive to loan only to qualified borrowers and to carefully monitor such loans. This decoupling of the local banks from local home buying led to new lending practices that have threatened the world economy. The increasing specialization of medical professionals might lead to a parallel crisis in medicine.

Perhaps one of the most powerful arguments that Dr. Gunderman makes is the need for medical schools to look beyond accumulated knowledge and IQ when they select new students. If medical schools ignore the emotional intelligence as well as the leadership characteristics of future doctors, they will create a medical profession that consists of brilliant technicians who don't understand and perhaps cannot even cope with the larger humanistic issues that are vital to the future of the profession. Let me be clear that this criticism is not specific to medicine. All the professions suffer from this same malady. Business schools and law schools are equally guilty of admitting technicians at the expense of generalists and need to take the same prescriptions that Dr. Gunderman recommends.

The concept of "ecotones" as discussed in his book is another interesting metaphor where the field of medical leadership can inform the field of leadership studies. In fact, this book itself represents an ecotone. Dr. Gunderman contends that "there are many ecotones in academic medicine." The same can be said of virtually all professions and organizations. For example, the leaders of the automobile industry would be well advised to consider the concept of ecotones in examining the rapidly evolving nature of their industry. Failure to do so could lead to failure of a number of the major automotive firms.

In his chapter on searching for a leader Dr. Gunderman makes the important, and typically overlooked, observation that the recruiting phase is perhaps the most critical phase for a new leader. It is during recruiting that the prospective leader has the power and flexibility to negotiate for the resources necessary to ensure the ongoing success of the organization. In fact, the failure to secure such resources during negotiations may be the single best signal that the position is potentially dangerous.

In sum, *Leadership in Healthcare* is a powerful treatise on the critical role of effective and enlightened leadership for one of society's most important professions. This is a book that should be read not only by leaders and aspiring leaders of the medical profession but also by scholars of leadership in general. The former will discover key insights from a wide range of disciplines that will inform their leadership practice and style. The latter will find a range of sometimes unique perspectives that can enlighten existing theories of leadership.

Philip L. Cochran

Acknowledgements

Numerous friends past and present contributed to my ongoing education in leadership and deserve thanks for helping to make this volume possible. I cannot catalog all the coaches and teammates, colleagues in fraternal, governmental, professional and civic organizations, coworkers in philanthropic initiatives, and members of faith communities who shared valuable leadership lessons. I first encountered leadership as a subject of study and practice through the Lilly Endowment Youth Leadership Program, under the far-sighted leadership of H. Dean Evans.

Many teachers have provided deep insights into leadership, most of which I only dimly recognized as such while under their tutelage. These have included, at Wabash College: Eric Dean, William Placher, Hall Peebles, Lewis Salter, and Raymond Williams; in the Committee on Social Thought at the University of Chicago: James Gustafson, Leon Kass, David Greene, Leszek Kolakowski, and Karl Weintraub; and in the School of Medicine at University of Chicago: John Fennessey, Thomas Krizek, Mark Siegler, Norma Wagoner, and Lawrence Wood.

More recently at Indiana University, Mervyn Cohen entrusted me with two leadership responsibilities that ignited a passion to begin studying leadership in earnest. Philip Cochran and Carol Madison in the Tobias Center for Leadership Excellence have permitted me to participate in a number of valuable leadership discussions and projects. In the Center on Philanthropy, Eugene Tempel, Dwight Burlingame, and Leslie Lenkowsky have done the same. Several people have made particularly important contributions to the School of Medicine's ongoing Leadership in Healthcare elective course, including Brandon Brown, Emily Beckman, and William Province. I also want to thank my regular conversation partners, William Enright, Paul Nagy, and Robert Payton, as well as Nancy Goldfarb and Richard Klopp. Thanks for Ruth Patterson and Rhonda Gerding for help in organizing my leadership teaching and preparing the manuscript.

Students and colleagues who have collaborated on prior work reflected in this volume include Shanaree Brown, Emily Burdick, Kenneth Buckwalter, Steve Chan, Nathan Erdel, Joshua Farber, Steven Kanter, Andrew Koerber, and Marsha Snyder. I would also like to thank several journal editors who have published some of my prior writings in this area, including Stanley Baum, Edmund Franken, Bruce Hillman, Anthony Proto, and Robert Stanley. Van Moore, Harvey Nieman, James Thrall and Christoph Wald have provided recent valuable opportunities to continue exploring leadership.

I would especially like to thank the many learners at the University of Chicago and Indiana University with whom it has been a delight to explore leadership over the years. Above all, my parents, James and Marilyn Gunderman, my beloved wife, Laura, and our children, Rebecca, Peter, David, and John, have taught me more than I can say about what a leader needs to be and do. Their love provides a wellspring of devotion and meaning on which it is a blessing to be able to draw each day.

Contents

Introduction

Let us begin with a story, a very unlikely story. A woman has two sons. As a matter of fact, they are twins. Her sons have grown into two very different young men, and she knows that only one of them is fit to carry on the family's enterprise and promote its larger mission in the community. Her enfeebled husband faces a dilemma whose significance he barely recognizes, the necessity of favoring one of his sons over the other in a way that both secures the family's mission and keeps it intact. Yet the father does not know his sons as well as his wife. He favors the lesser of the two, the firstborn, a jealous man who, if passed over, might resort to murder. Yet the mother knows that, should her husband choose the elder, all will be lost. Her husband's life, her sons' lives, and everything she herself has lived for will come to naught.

Of course, this is a very old story, from the Book of Genesis. It is the story of parents Isaac and Rebecca, sons Esau and Jacob, and the trans-generational covenant between the divine and father/grandfather Abraham. It is also an extraordinary tale of leadership that both anticipates and exemplifies many of the themes of this book. Its female protagonist, Rebecca, is a person who wields little authority and does not bear any formal responsibility for this momentous decision. Were we to inspect the organization charts of her culture and family, we would find authority bypassing her and flowing instead through her husband, Isaac the patriarch. Yet she does not resign herself or her family to a future of discord and lost opportunity. Instead Rebecca takes action.

The story leading up to this episode has established Rebecca as an extraordinary woman who might just make up for her husband's deficiencies. Decades before, when Abraham gazed on his unmarried son Isaac, he knew that he had to do something. His life purpose, the covenant, could be fulfilled only through his son and his son's sons. A wife had to be found for Isaac. Yet instead of sending Isaac, he sends a trusted servant back to his homeland to find a bride. Before departing, the servant says that he will know he has found the right girl when he asks for a drink and she draws water not only for him but also for his camels. When he arrives, the first girl he meets offers him water and proves the depth of her generosity by continuing to draw from the well until every one of his camels is sated. Her name, Rebecca, means "captivating."

After they are married, 20 years elapse before Rebecca finally conceives, recalling the infertility of Isaac's mother, Sarah. Rebecca's pregnancy is an extremely difficult one, and she senses that the two sons within her are constantly battling one another. From the moment they are born, they develop along two very different human paths. Esau, the firstborn, is a man's man, who lives for the hunt. Jacob, by contrast, is a homebody, perhaps even a mama's boy. While Esau spends his days out in the field hunting game, Jacob stays home and tends the kitchen. One day, when Esau returns from the fields empty-handed, he pleads with his brother for some soup, saying that he is at the point of starvation. Jacob agrees, but only on condition that Esau transfers to him his inheritance, the birthright of the firstborn. Esau, famished, readily agrees.

Later, the time has come for Isaac to bestow his blessing, the continuation of the covenantal relationship with the divine first undertaken by Abraham. According to it, Abraham and his progeny will produce many descendants who will enrich the lives of all the peoples of the earth. Isaac, whose vision has grown dim, prefers his elder son, Esau, who by birth-order tradition should receive both the birthright and the blessing. Hungry, Isaac sends Esau out into the field to hunt wild game and bring him some of the savory meat he loves, after which he will bless him. Overhearing Isaac's words, Rebecca calls Jacob to her side. She will prepare the meat, and Jacob, disguised as Esau, will take it to his father and receive the blessing. On hearing his mother's plan, Jacob objects, not because it is wrong, but because he is afraid that he will be detected and punished. Rebecca explains that she will disguise him to resemble his brother, saying she will bear all the blame. Jacob agrees, and brings his father the dish. Isaac expresses initial reservations, but eventually bestows a blessing on Jacob.

Later, when Esau returns, Isaac and he both realize with amazement what has happened. Esau is enraged, resolving to hunt down and murder his brother, reprising the original fratricide of Cain and Abel. Though mystified, Isaac refuses Esau's entreaties to retract the first blessing, instead bestowing on him a lesser one. Knowing what has transpired between Isaac and Esau, Rebecca hastily calls Jacob and tells him to go away to his uncle's house until his brother's anger subsides and she can send for him. In fact, Jacob will be away from home for more than 20 years, and these will be the last words Rebecca, who dies in the interim, ever speaks to him. She then tells Isaac that she could not bear for Jacob to follow his brother in marrying a foreign woman, and Isaac agrees to send him away to find a wife. Before Jacob goes, Isaac bestows on him a second blessing, this time the authentic covenantal blessing that his father gave him.

At first glance, the leadership lessons of this story seem to be cautionary ones, dramatizing the kind of conduct good leaders should avoid. In fact, most of my students initially regard Rebecca's conduct as reprehensible. How could she deceive her enfeebled husband and cheat her own firstborn son out of what was rightfully his? In fact, however, this story poses the essential questions of leadership, inviting us to look beneath the surface to find in Rebecca the marks of a great leader.

- From the first moment we meet her, we know Rebecca to be an extraordinarily caring and giving person. She is not scheming for her own gain, but working for the good of others. She helps those nearest and dearest to her see what they are called to be, creating circumstances in which they can fully express their latent virtues.

- Rebecca is faced with a seemingly insurmountable challenge: to preserve her family against destructive forces of jealousy and self-absorption, while at the same time enabling those she loves to discover and fulfill their proper roles. Lacking the formal power of patriarchal fiat, she proceeds by the only means at her disposal, guile. She foregoes knives for words.

- From the time her sons first moved in her womb, Rebecca has grasped their natures more deeply than their father. Esau the hunter is also a creature of the moment who willingly sells his inheritance for a bowl of soup. He lacks the long sense of time required of great leaders. Jacob, though a homebody, is capable of higher aspirations and able to view events from a longer perspective. He is the more fitting bearer of the covenant.

- Unlike her husband and eldest son, Rebecca does not operate from her belly. Instead, she operates from her head and her heart. Where others see only win-lose scenarios, she weaves a story in which everyone can fulfill his destiny. Her vision encompasses the entire family, including those who came before her (Abraham and Sarah) and those who will come after (Jacob, his wife, and their offspring).

- Rebecca confronts great hazards without losing her composure. She finds herself in a situation that offers no easy answers, asking her to strike a balance between multiple divergent, even seemingly incompatible ends. Yet she successfully negotiates the challenge by keeping her gaze firmly focused on the highest and best possible ends.

- Rebecca never loses hope. In the end, though she herself is no longer on the scene, her dreams are realized. Isaac finally realizes his true destiny and bestows the appropriate blessing on Jacob. Esau becomes a very prosperous and powerful man who, after more than two decades, eschews fratricide and reconciles with his brother. Above all, in the household of crafty uncle Laban, Jacob learns what it is like to be the victim of deception, eventually developing into a wise human being fit to bear the covenant.

One of the most remarkable features of this story is its steadfast refusal to provide easy answers, challenging us to find our own way in this complex human drama. Why wasn't Esau, the firstborn, the most fitting heir? Why couldn't Isaac see the true merits of his sons? Why didn't formal authority for these momentous decisions rest with the wisest and best person of the second patriarchal generation, Rebecca? If the purpose of human existence were to keep life as simple as possible and safeguard us against all possibility of error, then the world we inhabit would make no sense. But if life is about human choice and the development of our own capacity to choose, then the complexity of human affairs serves us quite well indeed. Rebecca's story is an invitation to explore and develop our own powers of discernment.

What if Rebecca is not deceiving Isaac but helping him see who his sons really are? What if she is not subverting the natural order but helping each of her sons see who he really is and who he is capable of becoming? By disguising Jacob she invites Isaac to look below the surface to their sons' characters. Which son is first, not by chance, but by nature? Likewise, she prods Jacob to consider what it would mean to be truly worthy of the blessing. By getting this homebody to take big risks, she helps him realize that survival and ease are not life's highest callings. Thanks to Rebecca, both Isaac and Jacob discover how to fulfill their destiny, realizing that they are called to serve purposes larger than themselves. What looks like base, self-serving deception is really a summons to self-discovery, self-actualization, and a shared sense of purpose. Rebecca is not a villain. She represents leadership at its best.

This volume on leadership operates in the shadow of this great literary tradition, one that puts questions before answers, character before rules, and persons before power. In healthcare today, with what covenants are we entrusted? Are we living up to them? How do we balance divergent and even conflicting missions? Is our horizon confined to the next quarter or the next annual report, or are we operating with a view to what our professions and our organizations will look like a generation or two from now? How well do we understand our colleagues and the people we serve, and to what extent are we helping everyone to realize their full potential? Do we have our priorities straight, ensuring that the lower, instead of subverting the higher, is always subordinated to it? How often do we pause to contemplate and discuss what matters most to us and the sacrifices we are prepared to make in the service of what is most important.

Like the story of Rebecca, this book is meant to be provocative, not definitive, and no reader will agree with every one of its contentions. It is not a how-to book on leadership or even an enumeration of the principles leaders should adhere to. There is simply no substitute for careful reflection and conversation about the challenges and opportunities before us, which are always too rich and nuanced to be captured by any manual. Instead this book consists of a series of essays, invitations to reexamine the kinds of choices each of us make every day. What we need above all is not more words of advice but opportunities to explore the moral dimension of leadership and prepare ourselves to make more insightful judgments. Techniques of leadership are less important than the philosophy of leadership. We need to nourish our moral imagination, enhancing our capacity to recognize not only problems with the status quo but also what could be and how we can bring it into being.

Medicine, nursing, and the other health professions need to invest more in such leadership development. Healthcare in the US is not well, and we have both a moral responsibility and a historic opportunity to play a leadership role in reinvigorating it and setting it on the right path. Yet health professionals have been playing a diminishing role in the leadership of healthcare organizations such as hospitals. The percentage of US hospitals led by physicians has fallen by 90% in the last three-quarters of a century. Physicians, nurses, and other health professionals have come to resemble Rebecca. Authority for policymaking in healthcare now largely bypasses us. Why?

We have allowed a powerful but incomplete model of physicians as purveyors of science and technology to overwhelm a more comprehensive vision of physicians as practitioners of the art of leadership. No one is suggesting that a renewal of physician leadership alone will cure what ails the US healthcare, or that every US healthcare organization should have a health professional at its helm. However, the need has never been greater for health professionals who know firsthand what it means to care for the sick to assume more leadership responsibility.

The greatest pathologist who ever lived, Rudolf Virchow, created the core medical lexicon we use everyday. He also offered a deep insight into what medicine really is. Virchow stated that medicine is not so much a biological science as a political science. By this he meant that it is not sufficient to understand biomolecules, cells, and organs. If we really care about health and disease, we must also understand the interpersonal, social, organizational, economic, political, and cultural dimensions of health and disease. It is not sufficient for the next generation of physicians to confine their attention to biological tools such as the microscope and the stethoscope.

We must also ensure that our successors know to how take full advantage of the tools of Virchow's political domain, including above all the hospital. Contemporary prejudices notwithstanding, hospitals are not businesses whose product happens to be healthcare. Patients are not mere customers, and physicians, nurses, and other health professionals not mere employees of healthcare vendors. Patients and physicians do not exist to serve hospitals and healthcare systems. Instead, hospitals and healthcare systems are tools that enable health professionals to provide patients and communities the best possible care.

Like Rebecca, we need to rediscover what is most important about the work we do every day, finding ways to help each of us do it better. In this spirit, the present volume is organized less like a pyramid than a tapestry. A pyramid is composed of independent, replaceable blocks stacked on top of one another, each occupying its own distinct space. By contrast, a tapestry is composed of innumerable threads, each interwoven with the others, the same themes appearing again and again in different contexts. Each thread is so intricately interwoven that it is difficult to tell where one ends and another begins. If we see but one thread of healthcare leadership, we do not see it at all. If we focus on how its many elements can fit together to form a mutually interdependent, coherent, and beautiful whole, we begin to understand what it is really all about.

Chapter 1
Why Leadership Matters

Physicians regularly face difficult choices. In the clinical sphere, we must detect subtle findings, determine whether an abnormality is significant, formulate a differential diagnosis, and conclude whether further evaluation is indicated. In academic medicine, we face choices between large numbers of candidates for admission to medical school and residency programs. Equally daunting is the choice of which research question to pursue. Some academic physicians are challenged to prioritize a variety of professional options, including direct patient care, research, teaching, and service. All physicians must balance personal and professional life, determining when the claims of work should take precedence over those of family, and vice versa. Making such decisions can be difficult, and professional training does not always prepare us to make them effectively.

The fields of management and leadership have responded to difficult decisions with quality movements, such as total quality management (TQM) and continuous quality improvement (CQI). In health care, these have helped departments, hospitals, and schools to better understand and enhance their work processes. Yet we need to shift our attention to even larger outcomes, such as whether particular tests and procedures actually improve health status, and whether their benefits are sufficient to warrant their cost. Health services research represents an effort to pose and answer these questions using reproducible observational and experimental methods. The bar has been raised, and mere case reports and clinical case series

R.B. Gunderman, *Leadership in Healthcare*,
DOI 10.1007/978-1-84800-943-1_1,
© Springer-Verlag London Limited 2009

no longer enjoy the same level of regard in clinical decision making as just decades ago. Instead of merely demonstrating that we have a new drug or device, we are challenged to show its value in improving outcomes or reducing costs.

The rise of scientific decision making represents a great boon to medicine, but it might easily become our bane. By focusing our attention on those variables that can be isolated and quantified, it may blind us to equally important factors that resist this approach. When we see only what we can measure, for example, we find ourselves blindly bumping into things we overlook – even really momentous things, like the meaning of our life and work. We need to remind ourselves from time to time that any theoretical framework necessarily simplifies a more complex reality, and something important can be lost in the process. A good theory helps us to discern the most important elements, but even a great one cannot capture everything. Focusing on any one factor necessitates the neglect of others. Astute decision makers study and utilize the best available models, but pause from time to time to check them against reality. The wisest among us know that discernment and common sense will never become obsolete.

Consider the evaluation of physical examination findings. Experienced physicians recognize the practical value of algorithms and heuristics. For example, it pays to have a system for assessing the lungs. Yet reliance on systems can sometimes compromise performance more than it improves it, in part because we tend to see what we look for. In Edgar Allen Poe's story, "The Purloined Letter," investigators fail to detect a letter resting on a writing table in plain view, because they operate from the assumption that it must have been cleverly hidden. Algorithms help us avoid overlooking aspects of a problem, but they are no substitute for stepping back and looking at it again from multiple points of view. Our theories show us some things, but they blind us to others. Truly great thinkers are able to shift back and forth between theoretical perspectives, occasionally inventing even entirely new ones.

Consider the daunting challenge facing admissions committees, which face a huge pool of qualified candidates. In an effort to be as fair and objective as possible, many committees rely heavily on quantitative indicators of merit, such as grade point averages and standardized tests scores. While such indicators offer advantages, they can also lead us seriously astray, if they become the sole basis of decision making. They do not encompass all of the personal characteristics that medical schools and residency programs need to consider. For example, they may underrate such traits as compassion and ingenuity. There is little evidence that they reliably predict future performance. And there is little or no evidence that programs that rely heavily on such criteria produce better physicians than those that do not.

Anyone who has ever read admissions essays or interviewed applicants knows that purely "objective" indicators are incomplete, at best. Some people who look very good on paper turn out to be less impressive in person. Some people with undistinguished academic credentials prove themselves capable of making substantial contributions in other ways. To perform well, we need to look beyond quantitative data and study personal essays and performance evaluations. A litany of scholastic triumphs can prove less salient than candidates' understanding of their own limitations, how effectively they learn from their mistakes, and what they are capable of imagining. It is important to be methodical, but we also need insight and creativity. We need to keep our eyes peeled for each candidate's distinctive genius. Relying on a rigid list of criteria can obscure some real gems.

The biggest problem confronting today's leaders is not the difficulty of weighing choices, but the failure to see the true range of alternatives. Some options are not mutually exclusive, and there are usually more than two options. Some of us get stuck in a rut, addressing each new situation in terms of long-established patterns. When your only tool is a hammer, the whole world looks like a nail. But we are never limited to just one tool. We need to open our eyes to the wider world around us. Some parts may respond well to hammering, but more will not. As Albert Einstein (Fig. 1.1) famously declared, "We cannot solve problems by using the same kind of thinking

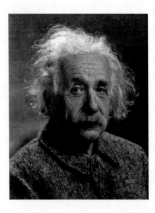

Fig. 1.1 Physicist Albert Einstein (1879–1955), who wrote, "We cannot solve problems by using the same kind of thinking we used when we created them." In a single miraculous year, 1905, Einstein, who was working full time as a patent clerk, published papers on special relativity, quantum theory, and other subjects that revolutionized theoretical physics, becoming the most important figure in the history of physics since Isaac Newton

we used when we created them." This is what it means to think "outside the box." Adaptability and innovation are every bit as important as reliability and rigor.

To think outside the box, we need to read and converse outside the confines of our discipline. Every field needs to participate in multidisciplinary, interdisciplinary, and even extradisciplinary conversation. Cross-pollination is an immensely powerful force. When it comes to expanding our field of vision, isolation is the enemy. The more we sit still, the further and further we fall behind. We need to look at what other people are doing and thinking from their points of view. Such perspectives help us to expand our sense of the possible, to see more clearly what we most heartily seek to accomplish, and to recognize the full range of resources we have at our disposal to help build a better organization. When it comes to effective leadership, conversation and collaboration are key.

***

Medical practices and hospitals spend great sums of money building and renovating facilities and purchasing new equipment, but relatively little time or effort developing a better understanding of the people who work in them. This practice overlooks a vital truth: organizations do nothing. It is not the organization, but the people who work in it that make things happen. Healthcare organizations can be only as good as their people. When something important needs to get done, the operative question is not, "Which button do I push?" but "With whom do I need to collaborate?" Healthcare leaders need to understand the nature of healthcare organizations and the work they do, and this means understanding physicians, nurses, technologists, administrators, and others who work in them. To improve organizational performance, we need to understand human performance.

This raises basic questions about the motivation to work. Are good workers born or made? Why do some people work harder and better than others? In hiring, can we predict which candidate is likely to do the best job? Are there steps leaders can take to enhance the motivation of the people they work with? What are the most effective motivators? Which is more effective, carrots, such as salary raises and public praise, or sticks, such as the threat of termination and reductions in compensation? Can we improve workers' performance through tighter control, or is it better to increase autonomy and empowerment? Most importantly, what can each of us do to improve our own commitment and dedication? Medicine's leaders cannot afford to neglect these questions.

If the people who work in healthcare organizations, particularly the leaders, do not understand the people we work with, performance will suffer. Organizations will experience difficulty recruiting and retaining employees, a prescription for disaster when key personnel are already in short supply. Work performance will suffer, compromising financial performance and endangering lives. Morale and commitment to the organization will suffer, because crucial needs and aspirations are not being attended to. Failure to understand human motivation hamstrings the organization. To foster greater dedication and fulfillment, leaders need to examine healthcare organizations in light of three twentieth century theories of professional motivation.

In his 1960 book, *The Human Side of Enterprise*, Douglas McGregor outlines two starkly different understandings of worker motivation. He argues that these divergent approaches to leadership grow out of two fundamentally different views of human nature, one negative and one positive. The negative one he refers to as theory X, and the positive one, theory Y. Leaders who favor authoritarian approaches and prefer to work in organizations with a high degree of centralized control tend to make theory X assumptions about human nature:

1. The average person dislikes work and attempts to do as little of it as possible.
2. People will work only if prodded into doing so through control, coercion, and threats of punishment. Otherwise, they will show little concern for the achievement of the organization's objectives.
3. People have little or no ambition, and wish to bear as little responsibility as possible. What they really want is security.

Leaders who operate according to theory X tend to be highly directive, telling workers what to do and involving them very little if at all in the decision-making process. When a worker asks, "Why do you want me to do that?" the answer is likely to be either, "Because I told you so," or "Because if you don't, I will punish you."

Theory X leaders are not interested in enhancing worker satisfaction and loyalty or helping workers achieve their ambitions, because they assume that they have none. They view the people who work in their organizations more or less as tools; useful so long as they can be made to do what is needed, but eminently expendable as soon as it becomes clear that they are not bending to the will of their superior. If a theory X health-care organization is to succeed in mission-critical tasks such as recruitment and retention, its leaders must either dangle very large carrots, such as exceptionally high compensation, or brandish very big sticks.

Theory Y offers a strong contrast to theory X, with much more positive assumptions about human nature. These include

1. Work is as natural to people as play or rest, and depending on the conditions, people may find their work a source of satisfaction and therefore want to perform it for its own sake.
2. External control and threats are not the only way to get workers to do what the organization needs. When people are committed, they will exercise self-direction and self-control.
3. People are more committed to organizational objectives that contribute to their own self-actualization, when they see their own achievement and that of the organization as intimately intertwined.
4. People not only accept but also actively seek out responsibility. If people avoid responsibility, display little ambition, and seem concerned only with security, it is generally because their work experience has taught them to do so and not because they were born that way.
5. The capacity to exercise imagination and creativity in the pursuit of the organization's objectives is widely, not narrowly, distributed.
6. In many organizations, the intellectual capabilities of the average person are only partly engaged.

In contrast to the authoritarian theory X leader, the theory Y leader attempts to create work conditions that match the needs and aspirations of workers with those of the organization.

Most physicians regard themselves as high achievers, and during their education grow accustomed to receiving recognition for their first-rate performances. Realizing this, a theory Y leader would look for areas of the organization in which each physician could make an important contribution for which he or she could earn recognition. A physician with a background in computer programming might be given responsibility and training to help implement a new hospital information system. Another with strong organization skills might be asked to design and implement a new faculty orientation and development program, intended to help faculty members reach their full potential by acquainting them with institutional resources helpful in their work. An overarching objective would be to involve colleagues in decisions about how their work is targeted, organized, and evaluated, always framed in terms of the larger strategic objectives of the department.

In broad terms, theory X presents a rather cynical view of human nature. It fosters the development of organizations that health professionals, who place a high premium on their own autonomy and self-direction, are likely to find stifling. Theory Y, by contrast, holds that the most effective way to run an organization is to respect and trust the people we work with, and above all, to work with them. How can leaders and prospective employees tell whether a department more closely approximates theory X or theory Y? We need but ask some simple questions: Do members of the department refer to its leaders by their first names? Do they get together on a regular basis to discuss departmental operations and strategy? Are they working together on projects? Do most members of the organization have special responsibilities in the patient care, research, or teaching missions? Do they refer to their work in terms of what they have been told to do, or in terms of their own initiative and participation on teams? Do they seem professionally challenged and fulfilled? Theory Y, not theory X, provides the better model for most healthcare organizations.

Psychologist David McClelland postulates that people have three fundamentally different sets of needs, which predominate to different degrees in different people. He emphasizes that these needs are not inborn, but are developed over time, depending on what sort of environment a person has been exposed to. While everyone has all three sets of needs to one degree or another, the set of needs that predominates in particular individuals can be expected to have a big impact on how we approach our work. These three sets of needs are

1. Need for achievement. This is the need everyone has to perform well relative to standards, to feel a sense of accomplishment in what we do, to help resolve problems, and to excel professionally.
2. Need for power. This is the need to influence or control how others behave and to exercise authority over them.

3. Need for affiliation. This is the need to be associated with others, to form and develop warm and friendly relations with one's coworkers, and to avoid conflicts.

Of the three sets of needs McClelland describes, the one that has received by far the most attention is the need for achievement. It should come as no surprise to physicians to learn that most of our colleagues feel a relatively high need for achievement. Understanding and tending to this need is a matter of particular importance for physician leaders. People with a high level of need for achievement tend to prefer situations in which we can take personal responsibility for solving problems. If we work in situations where we have little or no control over what happens, and therefore experience success and failure as though they were arising from chance, we are likely to become disaffected and lose motivation. Another characteristic of such people is a tendency to set moderately high goals for ourselves. We actually want to find projects that require us to exercise our full capabilities. If our position does not provide us with such challenges, we are likely to become bored and disengaged. Finally, such individuals want and need clear feedback on our performance. Our motivation will decline if there are no systems in place to help us assess whether we are achieving our objectives.

A second area of concern is the need for power. This need should be carefully attended to, particularly when selecting leaders and supervisors within the organization. It is important not to equate the need for power with a desire to control other people, or simply to be in charge. In its positive sense, the need for power reflects a sincere commitment to the success of the organization, and not merely a subterfuge whereby people use the organization as a means to our own self-advancement. People who seek power in this sense do so because we recognize that our influence over others can help the organization fulfill its mission. Such people want to have a positive impact on the organization and the people we work with. If the need for power is not attended to by an organization and people see we have no meaningful influence over its destiny, our need for power will go unfulfilled and we will look elsewhere for opportunities to play a more important role.

The third need, for affiliation, manifests itself as a desire to be identified with a group, and to be well liked by its members. People with a high need for affiliation may place a higher premium on the quality of relationships we enjoy than on our own accomplishments, and may prefer developing friendships to augmenting our own power. Such individuals may perform poorly as leaders. We want to be on good terms with everybody. As a result, we are unable to make tough decisions for the good of the organization for fear that we might offend some person or group of people. Discipline, enforcement of rules, and termination of employees are examples of situations that people with a high need for affiliation are likely to find troubling. As a result, many may find leadership positions frustrating, because we are regularly called upon to engage in activities that we instinctively avoid.

The relationship between the need for achievement and the need for power deserves special attention, particularly as regards the selection of leaders. People with a high need to achieve, though often the most successful people in a department, may not always provide the best leadership, and leaders should think twice about automatically appointing the best clinician, researcher, or educator to positions of authority. The success of the organization hinges on responsibility and control at the level of the group, not that of the individual, and this wider diffusion of responsibility and control may not suit some high achievers. In many situations, the more effective leader would be an individual with a high need for power, who naturally thinks in terms of the group and takes responsibility for what happens within it.

Business school professor Victor Vroom agrees that needs are extremely important in motivating human behavior, but argues that simply understanding what people need is not enough. In order to gain a complete picture of motivation, we must understand the factors that influence decision making about how needs will be satisfied. Vroom argues that there are three conditions under which this decision making takes place:

1. People must believe that making an effort will make our desired level of performance more likely. If we believe that we are unlikely to achieve the desired level of performance no matter how hard we try, we are unlikely to do so.
2. We must see how achieving that level of performance will help us realize some concrete goal or award.
3. We must value that goal or outcome.

Vroom adds to the other motivational theories the insight that people often view daily tasks not as ends in themselves, but as means to other ends. In other words, goals and achievements are not necessarily directly connected with one another, but may be separated by a number of intermediate links. He calls our assessment of the probability that our efforts will lead to a desired level of performance expectancy, while the probability that that desired level of performance will lead to the desired outcomes he calls instrumentality. Hence there are at least two levels of outcome, levels of performance and rewards. The first level of outcome, the effort to perform, includes parameters such as quantity or quality of work produced, attendance, and creativity. By contrast, second-order outcomes include earning the esteem of coworkers, the praise of supervisors, the ability to structure the work environment, and promotions. If we believe that our first-order outcomes do not contribute substantially to the achievement of our second-order outcomes, we are likely to perform at a lower level.

To expectancy and instrumentality, Vroom adds a third factor, valence. Valence describes the value that we attach to a particular outcome. For example, one individual might be relatively unconcerned about salary, in which case compensation would have a low valence, while for another person salary might be the most important feature of work, which would give compensation a high valence. Thus, a person could be absolutely certain that making a bigger effort would improve the quality of work (expectancy $= 1$) and that improved quality would increase compensation (instrumentality $= 1$), yet care very little about achieving a raise (valence = 0.1). Because the three factors are multiplicative, a lower value assigned to any one of the three factors leads to a low overall level of motivation. Leaders need to attend to all three factors if we are to help develop a work environment that fosters a high level of motivation.

The key for leaders is to determine what second-order outcomes really motivate employees. If the thing that motivates a group of physicians most is the compensation package, then an effective leader must find ways to enable them to augment their incomes by producing a greater quantity or quality of work. Conversely, if the thing that most motivates a group of physicians is the desire to make a significant contribution to the care of patients, then leaders must find ways to enable them to see the fruits of their patient care efforts. Alternatively, some physicians may place an especially high premium on expanding the envelope of medical knowledge through research. Others may prize most highly the opportunity to educate the next generation of physicians. Still others may find opportunities to make administrative contributions of greatest value. The key for leaders is to understand the people we are working with.

As McClelland indicates, however, these expectations are probably not set in stone and may be subject to environmental influence. Leaders should attend not only to what workers expect today, but also to the expectations of prospective employees, and to how everyone's expectations will be shaped in the future. These considerations vary depending on the nature of the organization itself. For example, in an academic department, it might be unwise to position compensation as the top second-order outcome, for fear that other academic missions such as research and education would soon be regarded as sources of inefficiency. In such a situation, the academic organization would either need to sustain lower-revenue-generating missions, such as teaching at the risk of losing workers to higher-paying clinical practices, or abandon them for the sake of generating even greater clinical revenues. In a practice situation specifically adapted to maximizing income, by contrast, such considerations would not obtain, and members could focus full attention on eliminating inefficiencies and maximizing throughput.

A final consideration is the fact that all persons in an organization do not necessarily share the same preferences regarding the rewards of work. The assumption that everyone is the same can prove disastrous. This is particularly true if new programs that appeal to the motivations of only a small number of people are applied across the board, as though everyone looked at work in that way. If an academic department decides to reorganize itself in order to maximize clinical revenues, yet this reorganization makes it increasingly difficult for devoted faculty members to find time to teach, then the educational mission of the department is likely to suffer, and educationally motivated faculty may choose to leave. The consequences of such decisions may take some time to fully emerge. Years might elapse before it becomes apparent that such a change in organizational philosophy is stimulating more residents to choose careers in private practice and contributing to a shortage of academic physicians. Leaders need to attempt to anticipate long-term effects of our policies, by adopting a longer-term strategic perspective.

There is no single, universally accepted theory of human motivation. Moreover, the three theories presented here barely scratch the surface of what is known. People and organizations are highly complex entities, and any effort to reduce motivation to a handful of factors is bound to produce some gaps and distortions. Yet this is no excuse for neglecting the subject. Medicine's leaders need to be scientifically knowledgeable and technically savvy, but we must also be people wise. The most important ingredient in the recipe for success is people.

Leaders must carefully explore who works in the organization, what working conditions the organization provides, and how these two interact with motivational factors to enhance or undermine the organization's mission. Do people have the ability to do what we need to do? Does the organization provide the resources we need to get the job done right? How well do motivational factors mesh with abilities and resources to make the organization a success? By understanding what makes people tick, leaders can do a better job of making our organizations hum.

***

Corporations that strive for high performance but invest little in their employees tend to perform well for only a short period of time. By contrast, companies that make big investments in their employees year after year tend to perform at a consistently high level. Taking good care of employees is not only ethically appropriate. It is also sound business. Consider the difference in return on investment between the average corporation and the Fortune magazine's "100 Best Companies to Work For." Between 1998 and 2004, $1,000 invested in the Standard and Poor's 500 would have grown to $1,387.70. By contrast, $1,000 invested in Fortune's "100 Best Companies to Work For" would have grown to $2,760.04. These represent overall returns over the 6-year period for the S&P 500 of 39% and for the "100 Best Companies to Work For" of 176%, more than four times better.

What are the key features of a great work environment? Three key ones stand out: trust, pride, and enjoyment. If we inspect medical practices and healthcare organizations in terms of these features, what do we find? How high is trust between physicians, nurses, hospital administrators, and other healthcare workers? Are colleagues proud of the work they do? Taking a friend or relative on a tour of the organization, would we be smiling and walking tall, or skulking about looking embarrassed? Day in and day out, do our colleagues enjoy their work? Do they see their role in the organization as more than a mere job? Is it a professional calling from which they derive genuine fulfillment?

Trust appears to offer a number of benefits. One such benefit is a tendency to promote high levels of collaboration. When people do not trust one another, cooperation and shared commitment suffer. Is a colleague out to usurp our job, or capture a promotion we are seeking? When such suspicions arise, we share less information. We keep to ourselves. We avoid collaboration for fear that it would undermine our competitive advantage. By contrast, when the level of trust is high, prospects for knowledge sharing are much more favorable. This promotes organizational learning. It enhances willingness to pool risks and resources in pursuit of a common goal. What risks are we willing to take for one another?

Building trust also fosters commitment. If an organization makes us feel like interchangeable parts in a machine, why should we feel any loyalty to it? If it relies on compensation to recruit and retain us, will we remain when better offers come along? We may even resent the organization, seeing the job as nothing more than a means of earning a living. When the work matters little, we invest little of ourselves in making it successful. Damage to trust foments turnover. How would we feel about a boss who operates according to rules like this: "Never fire employees on their birthday, anniversary, before a holiday, on a Friday, etc.?" It is like introducing your spouse by saying, "I would like you to meet my current husband (or wife)."

Trust also tends to improve customer support. If we feel trusted and genuinely committed to an organization's mission, we are more likely to go out of our way to take good care of patients. In a trusting environment, we see good service as an essential part of our own mission. When a problem or opportunity to improve arises, we do not dismiss it because it is not in our job description. Instead we seize it. In a healthcare organization, fear that infractions will be detected and punished is a less powerful motivator than a genuine commitment to provide the best care. Partnerships tend to be patient-friendly practice models, in part because everyone operates like an owner. We see our own interests as co-extensive with those of the organization.

Pride is another important feature of great organizations. If we are to perform at our best, we need to take pride in the work we do. Extrinsic aspects of work play a role. These include the quality of equipment, the general level of cleanliness and tidiness of the workplace, the prestige associated with the organization, and the level of compensation it offers. More important, however, are the intrinsic features of work itself. Are we and the organization doing our jobs well? Are we making an important difference in the lives of our colleagues, the patients we serve, and our communities? Are we improving the quality of work we do?

Consider a physician who publicly extols the importance of fostering collegiality and shared commitment, yet in private tends to refer to colleagues in rather disparaging terms, as though they were petulant children whose principal goal is to do as little work as possible. Instead of building pride in the organization, this individual foments an attitude of disdain and even contempt. As a result, when he attempts to build camaraderie and shared commitment, people doubt his sincerity. They feel patronized. They sense that he takes no genuine pride in their work, and this undermines his ability to lead. To build pride, we need to see the people we are helping. We need to develop real measures of quality and disseminate them throughout our organization. When we make progress in meeting them, we need to take the time to celebrate our successes.

The final major factor is enjoyment. For many people, the greatest barrier to enjoying work is not money. Highly educated professionals such as physicians rarely say that work would be more enjoyable if we made more money. The biggest barrier to enjoyment is time. Over the past few decades, US workers, including physicians, have been spending more hours at work and working harder while we are there. As productivity has increased, the enjoyment of those doing the work has been placed at increasing risk. We must not let the imperative to increase productivity undermine our ability to learn, to share experiences, and to develop and grow professionally.

Similar trends are evident in academic medicine. Many physicians choose academic careers because they enjoy research or teaching. We want to make a difference through research, education, and service. Yet as the clinical demands on our time continue grow, we find time for academic pursuits becoming scarcer. We begin asking ourselves why we remain in academic practice. Many choose to leave. If medical practices and healthcare organizations are to be good places to work, we need to make sure that our colleagues feel challenged by work, recognized for the quality of the work they do, and believe that through it they are growing as professionals.

Life is simply too short to carry on year after year in a work environment that provides no enjoyment and leaves us feeling cheated. Happily, a competitive market for labor tends to punish organizations that treat their workers like livestock, while it rewards good places to work. In the long run, organizations with low levels of trust, where people take little pride in their work and work itself provides little enjoyment, will suffer in morale, retention, and productivity. People tend not to care, and organizations pay a high price for it. It is not enough to offer higher compensation or more time off. The most discerning and capable physicians are not selling their services to the highest bidder. They are seeking out organizations that enable them to flourish as professionals and human beings. Organizations that cultivate trust, foster pride in work, and encourage physicians to enjoy what they do will enjoy immense competitive advantages and ultimately make a bigger difference.

***

Edward Gibbon's *The History of the Decline and Fall of the Roman Empire* has served as the foremost account of Roman history for over two centuries. Gibbon's work offers deep insights into timeless forces of dissolution that can undermine any large organization, including medical departments, group medical practices, hospitals, and even whole professions such as medicine and nursing. Some of these forces are evident today in contemporary health care. If we are to avoid following Rome's path to ruin, it is vital that medicine's leaders attend carefully to these lessons.

Edward Gibbon (Fig. 1.2) was born near London, England in 1737, the son of prosperous parents whose six other children died in infancy. At the age of 15, he entered Magdelene College, Oxford University, though he subsequently rued his time there as the most worthless period of his life. Gibbon spent his formative years in Lausanne, Switzerland, and after a period of service in the military, embarked on a grand tour of Europe. It was during his visit to Rome that he first conceived his great history of the Roman Empire, which would become perhaps the greatest work of history composed in the English language. The first volume was published in 1776, and the final ones reached the reading public in 1788. Gibbon also moved in elite literary circles and served in the House of Commons. He died in 1794.

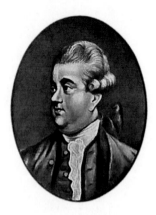

Fig. 1.2 Edward Gibbon, 1737–1794, author of *The Decline and Fall of the Roman Empire*, the first volume of which was published in 1776. This historical masterpiece provides a timeless reminder that even the mightiest of organizations are perishable and that failures of leadership often precipitate their demise

In its day, Rome represented the greatest political, economic, and cultural empire the world had ever known. From a small settlement on the banks of the Tiber River in 753 BC, by 116 AD it reached an area of over 2.5 million square miles, and dominated the history of Europe and North Africa for centuries. It produced great technological innovations in architecture and civic engineering, a stable system of government that kept the peace over a vast geographic and cultural range; great works of art including the epic poetry of Virgil, the histories of Tacitus and Plutarch, and the philosophical writings of Cicero and Seneca; and an unprecedented standard of living not equaled again in Europe until the seventeenth century.

Prior to Gibbon, historians commonly supposed that Rome fell because it was overwhelmed by external forces. The Huns, Goths, and Vandals swooped down on the Empire and vanquished its armies, eventually sacking the city in 455 AD. Rome collapsed, so the story went, because other cultures surpassed it, at least in terms of military might. In medicine, too, we sometimes talk as though barbarians are knocking at our gates, threatening to overwhelm us. These forces include declining payments for medical services, unsympathetic hospitals and healthcare corporations, and encroachment by rival providers who covet medicine's turf.

According to Gibbon, however, the fall of Rome should be traced not primarily to external forces. Instead the once seemingly invincible Roman Empire primarily decayed from within, which left it prey to outsiders. Had Rome not adopted self-destructive policies that weakened its own political and cultural resources, no external armies could have conquered it. The same can be said for medicine. The greatest threats to medicine are not external but internal, having to do with the decline of professionalism. Three of the most important lessons from the fall of Rome are: do not allow citizenship to degenerate into despotism, do not place increasing reliance on mercenaries, and do not become addicted to luxuries.

In the early centuries of Roman history, peoples who came under the rule of Rome enjoyed many benefits. The Romans had developed one of the most effective political systems in world history, with a constitution and a system of laws that were relatively fairly enforced. At Rome's apogee, politicians, magistrates, and soldiers saw the law not as a tool for their own enrichment but as a higher order to which they needed to subordinate their own appetites and ambitions. Citizenship in the republic was understood to entail duties, and fulfilling those duties was regarded a noble form of civic service and participation. Citizens saw paying taxes and serving in the military as privileges. Rome effectively united the freedom of popular assemblies with the authority and judgment of the senate and the executive powers of a fair magistrate.

The Romans did not view citizenship in exclusivist terms. They extended it to foreign peoples who spoke different languages, lived according to different customs, and even worshipped different gods. Instead of impressing conquered peoples into slavery, the Romans frequently invited them to join their ranks. They enjoyed huge benefits in enhanced public order and safety, economic enrichment, and cultural opportunities. Instead of building a fortress with ever thicker walls to exclude the barbarians, the early Romans built a tent of prosperity, and they kept expanding it to admit more and more peoples.

With time, however, Rome's republican form of government gave way to despotism. The senate yielded to the emperor, and relatively virtuous emperors such as Augustus were followed by dissolute successors. When Rome was ruled by the senate, lawmakers often thought first of the interests of the citizens, but later the ambitions of the emperor gradually took precedence. Corrupt emperors regarded senate and citizens as mere tools, worthy of attention only insofar as they could get the emperor what he wanted. Emperors concerned themselves less and less with serving the people, instead augmenting their own power and glory. In their eyes, a strong citizenry dedicated to defending the republic became a liability. They promoted policies that made the people progressively weaker and more dependent.

This attitude created enemies both inside and outside the Roman government. Within Rome, citizens become disenchanted. Instead of promoting the welfare of Rome, the emperors were manipulating the levers of government for their own satisfaction and aggrandizement. Foreign peoples under Roman rule began to regard the Empire as less a provider of opportunity than an oppressor. With time, this exploitation became intolerable to those laboring under the Roman yoke. Considerations of personal merit and justice had ceased to hold sway, and justice and liberty had been replaced by arbitrary despotism.

Something similar could happen in medicine. The health professions' strength lies in their ability to promote the best interests of patients, referring health professionals, and communities. At our best, health professionals make decisions about locating facilities, ordering tests, prescribing treatment, and providing service by putting the best interests of patients and the community first. The interests of health professionals come second. Medicine and other health professions can remain healthy only if we hold true to this professional mission. In the words of Confucius, "Those who seek the good of others have already secured their own." The corollary is equally straightforward: "Those who pursue only their own good are always undermining it."

If patients and the public sense that we care more about our own welfare than theirs and that we are using them as a mere means to get what we want, then we cease to be true professionals, becoming mere despots. It is impossible to trust people who use others as tools. It is impossible to feel loyal to people who see others as stepping stones to their own success. If medicine hangs its hopes on manipulating others for its own benefit, then it may go the way of the Roman Empire. The only way to secure the long-term future of any profession is to ensure that it makes valuable contributions to those it serves. The moment we begin to think of ourselves as the masters of those we exist to help, our moral authority begins to unravel.

Another lesson of Rome is the danger of relying on mercenaries. Throughout the early history of the Roman Empire, serving in the military was regarded as one of the most important responsibilities of citizenship. To most citizens, it was seen not as a nuisance but a privilege. Those who served regarded it as a badge of honor. Over time, however, the ideal of the citizen–solider eroded. Citizens ceased to see service as a personal responsibility, and preferred to pay others to do their fighting for them. They began outsourcing their own defense, become increasingly reliant on Barbarian soldiers of fortune. History reveals that such strategies work, if at all, only for a short time. Because mercenaries are not fighting for their homeland, they fight with less spirit. Motivated by avarice, some eventually turn on their employers.

The word mercenary derives from the Latin *merces*, meaning price. This is the source of our words mercantile and merchandise. It implies an overarching concern with wealth and profit, as opposed to honor. Mercenaries sell their services to the highest bidder, encumbered by no moral scruples about whose cause is just. To expect loyalty from a mercenary is to misunderstand what a mercenary is. They enter, exit, and reenter business relationships as needed to maximize their earnings. In the final analysis, they can be trusted to pursue but one objective: their own self-interest.

To what degree do physicians and other health professionals represent ourselves, and to what degree are we becoming increasingly reliant on outside consultants and lobbyists? To be sure, non-physicians with backgrounds in administration, business, and law make vital contributions to medical practices and professional organizations. Many physicians do not possess the requisite knowledge to ensure that our organizations perform at their best. Yet there is a big difference between hiring non-physicians to assist in navigation and turning over the helm to them. Physicians need to be engaged on the front lines of health care, building bridges and fostering collaborative relationships with patients, healthcare organizations, and communities. When we pay someone else to do it for us, we place our profession in peril.

What about medicine's academic missions? Are we providing future physicians with the knowledge and experience they need to perform well as biomedical investigators, or are we handing over the research initiative to non-physicians? To what degree are future physicians being educated to excel as educators in their own right, and to what extent are we ceding our educational responsibilities to others? Are physicians prepared and eager to play leadership roles in our healthcare system, or are we handing over such responsibilities to non-physicians? The Germanic mercenaries who came to dominate the Roman army eventually turned on Rome itself. What prevents medicine's mercenaries from turning on the physicians they were hired to support?

Another cause of Rome's decline and fall was a growing appetite for luxury. As the Romans grew wealthier, many citizens withdrew from civic life, spending progressively more time and energy on private pleasure. Keen to show off their riches, they eagerly sought out ever more ostentatious means of display. They installed baths, where prominent people basked in idleness. They constructed magnificent coliseums, which featured increasingly outrageous and brutal forms of entertainment. As time and energy shifted from civic engagement to private diversion, the quality of Roman civic life steadily eroded.

Declining civic engagement left the door open to tyranny. Occasionally, the monarch was a benevolent ruler such as Marcus Aurelius. More often, however, he was a despotic tyrant, who used the nation and its people as tools to satisfy his own appetites. Corruption became increasingly rampant, and people lost confidence in their system of government. Money supplanted merit, people were willing to sell their vote, and before long, whole elections were bought and sold. Long-term responsibility gave way to short-term expediency.

The same can happen in medicine. We can become so obsessed with money and the things that money can buy that we lose sight of the reason that medicine exists in the first place – to serve patients and communities. We find ourselves spending so much time thinking about the size of the house we live in, the features of the automobile we drive, or the tailoring of the clothes we wear that we allow teaching, research, professional and community service, and patient care take a back seat. We find ourselves putting our own interests first when we strike agreements with hospitals, healthcare corporations, and government. We cease to be self-regulating professionals devoted to higher purposes, becoming instead what Plato called "mere moneymakers," whose public virtues have been subverted by private vice.

The twentieth century abounds with examples. Consider, for example, the fate of many labor unions. During the second half of the century, membership in labor unions decline precipitously. Why? Many unions ceased to provide a sufficient level of service to their members. They developed a habit of caring more for their own staff than the workers they served. Likewise, they thought more about protecting the financial security of their rank-and-file members than about creating new jobs, helping to stimulate innovation, and meeting the needs of customers who bought their products and services.

Many unions fostered an us-versus-them mentality that emphasized winning short-term concessions instead of building long-term partnerships. Helping people to do good work became less important than preserving the status quo. Seniority supplanted excellence, and complacency overcame ambition. Job security was such an overriding concern that some union leaders thought it better to see workers get paid for doing nothing than to place any job at risk. As a result, everyone's jobs were placed at risk. Workers' commitment to innovation and flexibility was undermined, and the performance of unionized industries began to suffer. What happens to an industry where its long-term health becomes a secondary concern to its workers?

If medicine is to thrive in the coming years, we need leaders who understand well the lessons of Gibbon's *Decline and Fall of the Roman Empire* and put them into practice. We need to ensure that we never allow protecting our own income and making ourselves comfortable to trump the needs of patients and communities. An attitude of entitlement is anathema. We need to think first about what we can contribute, not what everyone else owes us. The healthcare system does not exist as a support apparatus for physicians, and our patients' diseases did not spring into being to provide us a livelihood. Our present convenience must never override the long-term missions of the profession.

We must keep our eye on our true mission. This is not filling out forms, analyzing data, or even collecting our paychecks. It is to use all the resources at our disposal to promote the interests of our patients and communities. Clinging tightly to the way we have always done things is not the best way to achieve this end. We need to play an active role in helping to improve medicine and the larger society in which it plays an integral role. Flexibility and innovation are key, and physicians need to position ourselves as visionaries, the shining examples of innovative leadership in health care.

Instead of building ever thicker and higher walls behind which to protect ourselves, we need to be reaching out and forging collaborations with others. Our value lies in building relationships with patients, other physicians and health professionals, and the communities we serve, striving to act as our communities' best citizens. Constructing an impregnable fortress leaves us completely isolated. Far from enhancing our security, a siege mentality would be our imprisonment, even entombment. We exist to make a difference in the lives of those who count on us. There are no barbarians at the gate.

Chapter 2
What Leaders Do

In order to excel at leadership, we need to know what leaders are and do. In this regard, examples of leadership in our popular culture may exert a powerful but unrecognized influence. Recent best-selling books on leadership have been read by hundreds of thousands and even millions of people, but portraits of leadership in novels, television, and cinema have reached audiences of tens or even hundreds of millions. Such portrayals shape our expectations of leaders and may ultimately prove more formative than formal leadership curricula. One of the greatest cinematic icons of our age is novelist Ian Fleming's signature character, James Bond. By examining Bond, we can gain deep insights into what leadership is and is not.

James Bond was one of the most popular literary and cinematic characters of the latter half of the twentieth century. Ian Fleming's franchise was so hugely successful that it carried on after his death by numerous authors, including Kingsley Amis and John Gardner. Over 20 major motion pictures have featured the Bond character, with more than a half-dozen actors playing the lead. The typical plot includes an ingenious villain, one or more vivacious female antagonists and accomplices, the legendary technoprops from Q branch, and of course, the various incarnations of the debonair Bond himself.

Bond is a cultural icon, as well known for his penchant for vodka martinis "shaken, not stirred" as for his espionage exploits. Few people are unfamiliar with "007," though many

R.B. Gunderman, *Leadership in Healthcare*,
DOI 10.1007/978-1-84800-943-1_2,
© Springer-Verlag London Limited 2009

may not know the meaning of the "00" designation: the agent's "license to kill" in performance of his duties. Bond films have been viewed by billions of people worldwide, and shape our vision of leadership in ways both subtle and not so subtle. This is not entirely regrettable, since Bond exhibits some desirable leadership characteristics. He is extremely clever and resourceful, he abhors cruelty, he exhibits a clear sense of purpose, and he is willing to take risks in performance of his duty. Yet Bond also exhibits many limitations and serves as a good illustration of a number of undesirable and even counterproductive leadership approaches.

In a representative Bond yarn, ordinary citizens are oblivious to the fact that a mad genius has concocted a diabolical plan to exterminate humanity and repopulate the planet with his own master race. The few world leaders who are aware of the plot hold out little hope of foiling it. Their only recourse is Bond. Notoriously contemptuous of bureaucracy, Bond chafes against the organization for which he works, MI-6, the British Secret Intelligence Service. Though he occasionally collaborates with other secret agents, such as Felix Leiter and Jack Wade, he is ultimately a loner. If espionage could be likened to musicianship, Bond would be an inveterate soloist.

What is the problem with Bond's individualistic approach? For one thing, it implies that leaders need to be heroes, ultimately relying on no one but themselves. When we hear the word hero, many of us think of military commanders, pilots, and sports stars, whose solo pursuit of excellence results in triumph. While other people stand about helplessly wringing their hands in despair, the hero swoops in, cuts through indecision and red tape, vanquishes the foe, and saves the day. Bond is so much the hero, the individualist, that it may be a mistake to call him a leader. His rank is commander, yet he rarely commands anyone.

As hero, a leader needs crises. Only during a crisis can heroism emerge. Where heroism is concerned, it is better to wait until the dam breaks and swoop in for a dramatic rescue than to prevent the disaster. There is no drama in dam maintenance. Yet making the leader's luminosity the principal concern undermines one of a leader's most important missions; namely, acting as a good steward of the organization. Creating situations in which heroes shine conflicts with the best interests of nearly everyone else. Crises are not the sign of good leadership. Quite the opposite, they usually represent failure.

It is counterproductive to pin our hopes on rescue. To do so is to fall into the trap of empty hope portrayed in Samuel Beckett's "Waiting for Godot." As expectations for rescue rise, our self-expectations fall. We begin to see ourselves as directionless, easily distracted, and inadequate. Anticipating a savior, we fail to seize opportunities to improve our situation ourselves.

Selecting a leader need not entail the forfeiture of our own initiative and commitment to collaboration. Seeing ourselves in the role of hero may lead us to underrate the initiative, ability, and leadership potential of our colleagues, treating them like defenseless sheep who must be rescued from a big, bad wolf. Our organization's vision, ingenuity, and perseverance are never confined to its titular leaders. We need a model of leadership that taps into the commitment and creativity of every member.

Does our model of leadership make passengers of us? On a bus, every person but one is a passenger, and only the driver has control over where the vehicle is headed. Our leadership model should more closely resemble an athletic team. On a team, success hinges on the integrated, second-by-second decision making of each player, all working toward a common goal.

What would it be like to work side by side with James Bond? Bond has no interest in collaboration. We slow him down, betray his presence, and botch his schemes. He works better without us. What does Bond want from us? The answer is simple: "Stay out of my way and you won't get hurt." True leaders bring out the leadership potential in each of us. They do not push us out of the way and make us feel worthless. They challenge us to contribute as much as we can. They do not merely bark out orders, but help us work together to develop and pursue a shared vision.

How does Bond see knowledge? He tells as few people as possible what he is doing. An informed person represents a security risk. It is difficult to know who can be trusted, and Bond is frequently betrayed by even his most intimate associates. Even those who would never willingly betray him may be duped or coerced into giving up sensitive information. And why should Bond tell anyone what he is up to, since in his mind he is the only person capable of accomplishing his objective?

In most Bond plots, the mission as originally presented to him by his superior, M, changes dramatically as he uncovers the true nature of the menace. Only Bond appreciates the full implications of the threat. He can engage in witty repartee with any number of clever people, but there is no one he can really talk to. He keeps all his cards close to his chest. The world of the secret agent is grounded in secrecy.

From the standpoint of healthcare organizations, secrecy is poisonous. We need to foster openness and knowledge sharing. Each of us needs to see what we do in the larger context of what others are doing. The key word is not heroism but collaboration, or better yet, synergism. We need to build teams.

Leaders need to think less about saving the day and more about promoting the long-term flourishing of organizations. To do that, we need to understand who we are, where we have come from, and where we are headed. Unlike James Bond, we cannot afford to operate strictly in the present, responding only to the pressing concerns of the moment. We need an outlook that is not only tactical but strategic, focused on developing our capabilities for the long term.

In the real world, no one has all the answers. We need to share knowledge and work together to solve problems. When we inform leaders of problems, we should not expect to drop them on their desk, turn around, and leave. Instead, we should expect to play an active role in helping to solve them. Likewise, when colleagues bring us problems, we should invite them to participate in finding solutions.

Bond films also contribute to the misapprehension that life is a battle between good and evil. In Bond, there is always a clearly identified villain, sometimes an operative of SPECTRE or SMERSH, but more often a solitary megalomaniac, such as

Dr. No or Auric Goldfinger. Every Bond drama is a clash between white hats and black hats. In the real world of contemporary health care, by contrast, there are no good guys and bad guys. In one way or another, everyone is trying to do a good job. It is vital that we resist the temptation to picture others in black hats, merely because their plans do not conform to our own. Instead, we should get to know them better, try to understand more clearly what they think they are doing, and work with them to develop a shared vision for the future.

Such conversations occasionally reveal unexpected opportunities for mutually beneficial collaboration. The good guy–bad guy mindset leads to win–lose scenarios, where we act with the misguided conviction that our success requires the other's failure. No good leader carries a license to kill. Instead of live–die or win–lose situations, our goal should be to create scenarios that are live–live and win–win. By helping others thrive, we are more likely to thrive ourselves. Bond makes an entertaining hero, but we need leaders who truly lead.

***

For insights into the nature of leadership, we could hardly turn to a better source than one of the greatest minds in the history of western civilization, Aristotle (Fig. 2.1), who lived in the fourth century BC. His range of interests included astronomy, economics, ethics, logic, metaphysics, meteorology, physics, poetics, politics, psychology, rhetoric, theology, and zoology. His works in these areas rank among the most important ever produced. In some notable cases the subjects themselves were not even recognized before he wrote on them. While Aristotle devoted most of his energies to what today we call philosophy and natural science, playing little direct role in politics himself, we are fortunate that his philosophical legacy includes many insights on leadership.

Aristotle famously wrote in the *Politics* that "Human beings are by nature political creatures." We naturally come together to form associations of one kind or another, and it is impossible for us to develop into the kinds of creatures we are intended to be absent a community. However, the state exists for the good

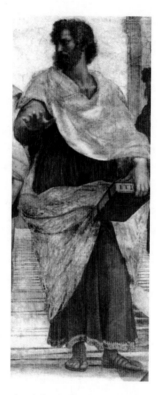

Fig. 2.1 Detail from the *School of Athens* by Raphael depicts Aristotle (384–322 BC), bearing a copy of his *Ethics* in one hand, his other hand outstretched in a gesture toward the world around us. A master student of the natural sciences, social sciences, and humanities, Aristotle's influence over the course of intellectual history has been incalculable

of the citizenry, not the citizenry for the state. Again in the *Politics*, he wrote "A state is not a mere society, having a common place, established for the prevention of crime and the sake of exchange. Political society exists for the sake of noble actions, and not of mere companionship."

The state is a means to promote an even greater end; namely, the flourishing of the people. For the people to flourish, we need to be properly reared and educated, and to enjoy opportunities to cultivate our excellences. Aristotle recognized many different types of excellence. These include bodily excellences such as good health, strength, and beauty; moral excellences, such as courage, moderation, and generosity; and intellectual excellences, such as cleverness and wisdom.

He recognized that all human beings are not equally equipped to lead. For example, some people lack the requisite mental capabilities. Others with real intellectual gifts lack interest in playing a leadership role, preferring instead the strictly contemplative life of study and writing. Others lack the interpersonal gifts that leaders rely on. Still others, the best candidates for leadership, possess the requisite intellectual and interpersonal gifts, as well as the necessary interest in public affairs and personal ambition, to excel as leaders.

Aristotle held that the highest offices in an organization or community should be filled by the people with the greatest abilities. He writes in the *Politics* "They should rule who are able to rule best." When inferior people are in charge, everyone, including the inept leaders themselves, will suffer their shortcomings. Hence it is important that organizations create leadership development opportunities for our most gifted people. If such opportunities are not available, talent, one of the organization's most precious resources, will be wasted. Those whose abilities are not engaged may grow disenchanted and flee or rebel.

Aristotle asserts that people need to have a stake in our organization or community. This investment may take the form of property or time and energy. People who hold such a stake will be better suited to lead because our vision of our own interests will be more closely aligned with the common good. People without such stake may become apathetic, or our interests may diverge so greatly from the needs of the organization that we end up opposing its interests.

Aristotle naturally viewed tyranny with skepticism. In the ancient Greek context, a tyranny is an organization in which all power rests with one person. To maintain power, tyrants usually suppress the development of others' abilities because they pose a threat to autocratic authority. In terms of the organization's best interests, such suppression is imprudent because it deprives the organization of the contributions of its most capable people. It is also unjust because it does not allocate responsibility in a manner commensurate with ability. Tyrannies are necessarily short lived, and the only stable state is one in which all men are equal before the law.

Another problem with tyranny is transition. No individual can govern forever, which raises the question, who will replace the tyrant? Hereditary succession is fraught with peril. The histories of monarchies throughout the world attest that even the most excellent leaders do not necessarily produce good offspring. The tyrant's intrinsic jealousy stunts the development of worthy successors.

Aristotle believed that relatively few people are cut out for high leadership positions. A flourishing organization or community has a great interest in ensuring the full development of every one. Recognizing that groups typically outperform individuals, Aristotle believed in the power of collective understanding. In a group, each member brings to the table different insights and experiences, providing a greater range of perspectives on a problem than any single individual.

Encouraging the members of an organization to play an active role in its affairs invites each of us to develop more of our potential. The founders of the United States, strong proponents of democracy, did not for a moment suppose that the citizenry would never make mistakes. They grasped better than any legislators in human history the significance of human fallibility, and they developed a system of checks and balances between the legislative, executive, and judicial branches of government. Yet they also believed in government by, for, and of the people. Many citizens could sustain a more just and stable government than a few powerful rulers. As Tocqueville pointed out, government by the people makes the governors more responsive to the needs of the governed.

Democracy requires active participation and that participation cultivates the very excellences necessary for citizens to flourish as human beings. Trials by jury do not always produce just decisions, but they do foster the civic virtues of the people who serve. By encouraging people to play an active role in governance, Aristotle believed, we help them to become better informed, more responsible, and more engaged members of the organization. As he writes in the Politics, "If liberty and equality are chiefly to be found in democracy, they will be best attained when all persons alike share in the government to the utmost."

Another advantage of political participation is the fact that it promotes commitment to democratically developed policies. People who have no voice in framing priorities generally feel little commitment to them. A policy need not be one with which everyone agrees. Some may have argued against it. Yet the fact that everyone's views received a full hearing, and the belief that the policymaking process is fair, tends to promote loyalty to the organization. One of the surest ways to promote dissension and revolt is to take away the opportunity for free discussion or to deprive people of suffrage we once enjoyed.

To highlight another advantage of participative governance, Aristotle points to the example of a house. Who is best qualified to judge the quality of a house, the person who built it or the person who lives in it? The person who built it knows a lot about its design and construction, including many features that the homeowner probably does not recognize. Yet the purpose of the house, ultimately, is to serve as a residence, not an opportunity for self-expression by the builder. The resident is best equipped to evaluate how well the house is performing, and what might be improved.

The same might be said for any system of governance. Those in charge may know a great deal, but frequently they cannot see the organization from the members' point of view. People may refrain from sharing bad news with leaders, for fear their career will be adversely affected. Leaders may spend little time with colleagues because they believe they have more important things to do. This can leave the leader out of touch and unable to lead effectively. It is vital to encourage regular and frank dialogue within organizations, so that leaders can adjust according to the views of those they serve.

Medicine can achieve its missions only with the collaboration of healthcare organizations, and the quality of organizations it helps to build will determine its future. As Aristotle reminds us, the best organizations are ones that see themselves as engines of human flourishing.

***

The performance of medical practices and healthcare organizations is a product of two key factors: the people who make them up, and the form in which they are structured. Even organizations made up of the very best people may perform poorly, if they are organized in ways that pit people against one another or prevent them from working together productively. Conversely, even organizations that are perfectly structured may not perform well if the people who occupy key positions are not well suited to challenges. This discussion focuses on the second of these key performance parameters, organizational structure. It draws heavily from the work of the one of the most influential contemporary organizational theorists, Henry Mintzberg. Mintzberg's taxonomy of organizational forms provides a theoretical scaffolding for leaders who seek to understand the impact of structure on organizational performance. He describes four basic organizational forms. These are the machine bureaucracy, the entrepreneurial startup, the professional organization, and the "adhocracy."

Each of these organizational forms is found in a distinct setting, according to two key environmental factors: the degree of environmental complexity and the pace of environmental change. Machine bureaucracies are found in stable environments where the level of complexity is low. Entrepreneurial startups are found in environments where the level of complexity is low, but the pace of change is rapid. Professional organizations are found where the environment is stable, but the necessary level of organizational complexity is high. Finally, adhocracies are found in environments where the pace of change is rapid, and a complex organization is required. By examining each of these forms and its distinctive strengths and weaknesses, healthcare leaders can better understand and improve the performance of our organizations.

In a machine bureaucracy, the organization emphasizes the standardization of procedures and outputs. It is dominated by technocrats, who apply their expertise to ensuring that members of the organization produce a prescribed product in a prescribed way every time. The organization is dominated by rules, standardized operating procedures, routines, and regulations. If we need to know what to do in a particular situation, we should consult a policy and procedure manual or its equivalent. In such organizations, decision-making authority tends to be relatively centralized, and most workers basically do what they are told. Typically, there is a sharp distinction between the people who are producing the product and the people who supervise them, with clear delineations between different levels of rank and decision-making authority. The key parameter of a machine bureaucracy is efficiency. We know what we need to produce – our product – and the priority is to do so with as little waste as possible.

Is machine bureaucracy an appropriate model for a healthcare organization, such as an academic department or a national organization? This model can function well only where the environment is relatively static, and the level of organizational complexity required is low. Before allowing such a structure to emerge, however, leaders should verify that our organizations have changed relatively little in the past few years and are unlikely to need to change substantially in the foreseeable future. Moreover, we should ascertain that a relatively simple organizational structure is adequate to meet the challenges facing the organization.

This form of organizational structure is poorly adapted to environments that are changing rapidly. It does not make sense to focus on producing ever better buggy whips at an ever lower per-unit cost if the transportation industry is in the midst of a transition to the horseless carriage. Similarly, the simplified command and control structure of a machine bureaucracy, in which all decision-making authority rests with a few people who tend to be far removed from the "front lines" of production, tends to perform poorly when confronted with new challenges. Given the increased levels of organizational complexity and the rapid changes taking place in the healthcare environment today, the machine bureaucracy is unlikely to be the best organizational structure for most healthcare organizations.

The entrepreneurial startup differs dramatically from the machine bureaucracy. There are no elaborate policy and procedure manuals. There is no command and control mechanism to keep precise tabs on what everyone is doing. The division of labor is not rigidly and precisely specified, and the managerial structure, if one exists, is likely to be small and loose. There is no elaborate strategic planning process, and people generally train for their work "on the job." The organization does not exhibit multiple levels of bureaucracy, and many individuals report directly to the leader, who is generally also the founder. Such organizational structures are most common in the early, formative years of a new organization. Yet many organizations continue to operate successfully in an entrepreneurial startup mode for decades. So long as the core leadership of the organization remains sufficiently dynamic, it can continue to grow and adapt to a changing environment. Many machine bureaucracies eventually fall prey to entrepreneurial startups because they are not nearly as nimble or creative and cannot recognize and respond effectively to new challenges or capitalize on new opportunities.

If such organizations do not eventually evolve beyond a startup mentality, however, they typically run into trouble when the founder dies or leaves the organization. A machine bureaucracy can easily tolerate the loss of a leader, but an entrepreneurial startup may be devastated. Some departments have performed well under the leadership of an outstanding chairperson, only to falter after the individual's departure. For this reason, organizations need to invest in the diffusion and development of leadership capabilities, so that they never become wholly dependent on any single person or small group of individuals. The best leaders resist the temptation to make ourselves indispensable, and instead cultivate the leadership capabilities of others. In effect, we are always training our successors. Such training can only take place in organizations that are structured to provide junior people the opportunity to shoulder real responsibility. For example, a department with a strong executive committee, made up of highly motivated and talented individuals, can carry on even after a great chairperson has departed.

Is the entrepreneurial startup the right model for most healthcare organizations? Probably not. For one thing, most organizations have been in existence for decades and have already undergone numerous leadership transitions. Founders are rarely on hand, and entrepreneurship is not the word that characterizes the attitudes of many hospitals and medical schools. The entrepreneurial spirit is also curtailed by the fact that most medical departments are situated in larger hospital and medical center bureaucracies, which may constrain innovation and foster an attitude of conservatism. Often more time and energy are invested in preserving the status quo than in spurring change.

Many medical organizations bear a closer resemblance to professional bureaucracies. A professional bureaucracy relies on an elaborate system of training and indoctrination to endow individuals with a strong internal compass, then allows us a great deal of control over our own work. In medicine, this training system tends to be prolonged and intense and includes medical school, residency, fellowship, and continuing medical education. As a group, professionals strongly value our own autonomy, and generally avoid stepping on one another's toes. On the other hand, we often interact very closely with the clients (patients) we serve. In a professional bureaucracy, standards of quality are enforced not primarily by external oversight, but by very strong internal expectations. Professionals police ourselves to ensure that standards are not breeched. Attempts to impose external control tend to be resisted, on the grounds that no other group possesses sufficient expertise to evaluate the profession's members. Such organizations tend not to be directed by a central overseer, but by the cumulative effects of individual members' aspirations.

Professional bureaucracies can function effectively so long as their environments are not experiencing rapid change. Provided that members of the professional bureaucracy clearly understand our respective roles, and so long as we do not need to engineer fundamental changes in how we operate, incremental adaptation may suffice. Yet in situations where rapid adaptation or innovation is called for, they are liable to perform poorly. When confronted by new competitive threats from other more dynamic organizations, their innate preference for stability often proves a serious liability. The professional bureaucracy responds to change not in a revolutionary fashion, but in an evolutionary fashion. Mintzberg suggests that substantial changes can require a generation or more to complete.

Healthcare organizations need to strike a balance between being swept up by every gust of change and stubbornly clinging to the way things have always been done. One strategy by which professional bureaucracies can respond to the need for rapid adaptation is to create project groups or task forces that can operate outside the usual bureaucratic box. If medical practices and healthcare organizations strive to preserve and promote a professional heritage, such as a time-honored code of ethics, they may function quite effectively even in the midst of change. On the other hand, this model is not optimally suited to creating and seizing new opportunities.

The inspiration behind project groups is embodied in the organizational form for which Mintzberg evinces the greatest enthusiasm, the adhocracy. Derived from the Latin phrase ad hoc, "for this," adhocracies rely on small groups that come into being to tackle specific tasks. Such groups are the antithesis of standing committees, whose standardization and routinization foster bureaucratic stagnation. In contrast to bureaucracies, the membership rosters of adhocracies tend to be both informal and interdisciplinary. They cannot rely on a command and control model of authority because the same group of individuals – such as a departmental executive committee or the board of governors of a professional association – does not enjoy sufficiently broad expertise to tackle every problem.

The emphasis in adhocracies is on problem solving, not on efficiency. Such organizations continually seek out new ways of doing things. They avoid a silo mentality in which different specialists and different divisions segregate knowledge from one another. Such compartmentalization prevents the interdisciplinary and interdepartmental exchange on which organizational creativity depends. No single person knows enough to excel at everything. The key to solving problems and creating new opportunities is getting people together to share problems and perspectives.

Adhocracies are well positioned to flourish in situations where change is rapid, and a complex organization is required. Project teams continually adapt their own and one another's outlooks to the opportunities before the organization. With this advantage comes a pitfall. Adhocracies tend to place a great deal of pressure on people to keep innovating and adapting all the time. People may feel that we can never simply kick off our shoes and get comfortable with the status quo. On the other hand, dynamic and enterprising people may thrive in these environments. Such individuals are continually on the lookout for challenges that enable us to grow and develop, and this vigilance invigorates us. We are more afraid of stagnation than change, and such enthusiasm can prove infectious. Even large and very complex organizations can function as adhocracies. If they manage to do so, they may retain much of the nimbleness usually associated small start-ups. They can create better learning environments than other organizations and do a better job of putting these lessons to use for the organization's benefit.

Is the adhocracy an appropriate model for healthcare organizations? It is probably inappropriate for entire departments or national professional organizations to adopt such forms, in part because adhocracies work best focusing on particular missions, not as administrative umbrellas. However, most organizations could attempt to exploit the distinctive strengths of adhocracies by creating interdisciplinary working groups to tackle particular problems and opportunities. If such groups are to succeed, however, they must enjoy real responsibility and real authority and have at their disposal the resources necessary to meet their charge.

For example, a department might appoint a small group of individuals to solicit advice, plan, implement, and evaluate a new information system, or a national organization might appoint a task force to develop a proposal to address rising healthcare costs. A small group working on a specific challenge can often achieve better results than a large group with many items on its plate. If adhocracies are to succeed, however, the leaders of the parent organization must resist the temptation to micromanage their work. We can observe and perhaps even participate in their deliberations, but we should not seek to dominate them.

Healthcare organizations and the people who lead them need to understand different organizational forms and their distinctive strengths and weaknesses. The performance of even the best people will be constrained if their organization is not appropriately structured to meet the challenges before it. By contrast, if an organization is able to adopt a structure that fits its needs and opportunities, the prospects for success become considerably brighter. In this respect, good leaders are like architects, attempting to achieve a union of structure and function. Achieving the appropriate organizational form depends on what the structure is intended to do.

Chapter 3
What Leaders Know

W. Edwards Deming once wrote that learning is not compulsory, but neither is survival. Physicians can be the best lesion detectors and differential diagnosticians in the world, yet if medical practices and healthcare organizations perform poorly, medicine will fail to deliver. The degree to which medicine prospers professionally, intellectually, and socially is determined in large part by the flourishing of the organizations that comprise it. This means that we need to cultivate the organizational expertise of physicians, and in particular, the ability to learn. During the twentieth century, most important insights into the structure and function of organizations originated outside of medicine, in fields such as business, history, and sociology. To secure medicine's future, physician leaders need to look beyond the curricula of medical schools and explore what makes organizations thrive.

Leaders need to cultivate organizations' ability to benefit from their own past experiences. As Peter Senge has emphasized, we need to build learning organizations. Organizations that fail to learn perform below their potential and are soon surpassed by the competition. Organizations that learn effectively enjoy an immense competitive advantage. How can healthcare leaders prepare organizations to learn more effectively? This discussion examines three models of organizational inquiry. These models are known as action science, action learning, and after-action review.

The model of action science is closely associated with the work of Chris Argyris and Donald Schön. As an approach to

R.B. Gunderman, *Leadership in Healthcare*,
DOI 10.1007/978-1-84800-943-1_3,
© Springer-Verlag London Limited 2009

organizational inquiry, it focuses on identifying and over-
coming obstacles to organizational innovation. Organizational
inquiry is based on the premise that organizations can improve
their effectiveness. If an organization is already as good as it
can possibly be, then no organizational theory will benefit it.
To organizations that have room for improvement, however,
action science has something to offer. The potential benefits are
greatest in the area of non-routine and particularly challenging
problems and opportunities.

Action science draws a fundamental distinction between
model I and model II theories of action. A model I approach
to organizational inquiry represents a simplistic but quite per-
vasive view. It states that it is up to leaders to define and pursue
goals and to direct colleagues in achieving them. On this model,
the leader designs and implements the organization's strategies
and action plans. Everything that happens in the organization
is a product of the leader's will. Where risks are involved, it is
up to leaders to protect the organization. The leader who
defines whether or not others are doing a good job, and everyone is expected to respect and abide by the leader's assessment.
Model I theories bear a strong resemblance to what have been
called "command and control" styles of leadership.

What happens when an organization is dominated by a model
I approach? Generally speaking, trust suffers, and people act
defensively to protect their own interests. Innovation is stifled
because people feel inhibited about sharing knowledge and
taking risks. In model I organizations, there is a strong emphasis
on competition. New people quickly learn to avoid certain
disaster – opposing the leader or making mistakes. We aim to
conform, to fit into the leader's vision. The level of intrinsic
commitment to the organization and its strategies is low because
people rightly feel that we have no role in helping to shape them.
Very little learning takes place, and the organization tends to
stagnate over time. The model I organization is a dinosaur
awaiting extinction.

By contrast, a model II approach gives people a much greater
role in helping to shape the organization, increasing intrinsic
motivation to move it forward. It places a high value on

discovery and knowledge sharing, as well as individual initiative and autonomy. Because people have access to more knowledge and can make better-informed choices, the quality of decision making is higher. In contrast to command and control leadership, model II leaders function in a much more participatory mode, empowering colleagues to do our best, and rewarding good performance with more responsibility and authority. Compared to a model I organization, a model II organization is a somewhat riskier but much more rewarding place to work.

In contrast to the competition of model I organizations, a model II organization fosters collaboration. People are less defensive because we have less to fear from one another and more to gain through mutual engagement. The general level of trust is much higher. When disagreements arise, people feel free to share viewpoints openly, knowing that our perspectives will be taken seriously and judged on their merits. When leaders express an opinion, we expect it to be carefully evaluated, not swallowed whole merely because it emanates from a position of authority. It may appear that there is more dissension in a model II organization, but the deeper reality is a livelier level of organizational dialogue. The quality of understanding in the organization is higher, and as a result, the long-term effectiveness of the organization is enhanced.

The learning that goes on in a model I organization is said to be "single-loop learning." People are so afraid of being shown up or embarrassed that we generally avoid addressing the underlying causes of our own discomfort. We would rather avoid problems, or at least avoid recognizing them, than confront them. The standard approach is simply to deny that problems exist. If problems do manage to come to light, people seek a way to ignore them. Model I is poisonous to organizational inquiry and undermines organizational learning. In the short term, it can be more comfortable because it avoids certain kinds of tension. In the long run, however, it dumbs down the organization and renders it vulnerable to competitors who take learning seriously.

Model II asks tough questions. How are we doing? What are we doing? Are we doing the right thing? How do we know? In other words, model II opens up both the organization's effectiveness in achieving its goals and the very goals the organization is pursuing. Because the healthcare environment is constantly changing, our outlooks need continual scrutiny and revision. No single organizational structure will suffice forever, and we need to regularly question and re-question what the organization is doing.

Another approach to organizational inquiry is action learning. It was developed by Reg Revans in England and came to prominence in the United States largely through application at the General Electric Corporation. Action learning puts a group of people to work on a real-life problem, then fosters reflection on how lessons learned can be applied to benefit each member, the group, and the whole organization or field. The technique is useful for strategic planning and tactical problem solving, for formulating a mission statement, and for creating a climate more favorable to inquiry and organizational learning.

It is important that groups work on real problems, not hypothetical ones. The problem should be a challenge or opportunity that all members of the group have a stake in. Finding a solution should be a high priority for everyone involved. Ideally, the problem should also offer cognitive leverage, that is, the lessons learned in working on the problem should be useful in solving other problems in the future. It should also provide an opportunity to educate people, allowing us to develop knowledge and skills that we can put to good use in other contexts.

The group itself should be small, fewer than 10 people, and include a variety of perspectives. Diversity must be a high priority. It does little good to assemble a learning group when people are carbon copies of one another. Such a group has little chance of outperforming its individual members. People need to listen to one another not only respectfully, but with genuine curiosity about other points of view. No one should operate with the presumption that there is a single right answer. The focus should be on formulating the problem as clearly as possible. Like Socrates, action-learning theorists prize asking the right questions more than to finding the right answers.

The members of the learning group need to embody a real commitment to inquiry. If people merely go through the motions to please a colleague or superior, little insight will emerge. More important than solving the problem at hand is developing intellectual capital, on which the organization can draw again and again. Such capital is not worn out or used up. It is augmented by repeated use. One way to promote engagement is to ensure that members' recommendations are discussed and acted on by the organization. Better yet, group members can be given authority to implement their findings and assess the results. The primary goal, however, is always to learn.

A famous equation associated with action learning is $L = P + Q$. L stands for learning, P for programmed knowledge (what the group already knows), and Q for questioning insight. Based on this equation, what a group is capable of learning hinges to a substantial extent on what it already knows. This helps to explain why it is important to populate groups with diverse members, whose combined knowledge exceeds that of any individual member. It also explains why action learning offers such important long-term benefits to the organization. As new knowledge and skills are developed, each subsequent action-learning opportunity takes advantage of a larger base of programmed knowledge. Yet past learning is not enough. The group must also ask new questions that lead to new insights.

The learning that takes place in action learning is highly experiential. Group members are not simply looking for answers to problems in textbooks or journals, nor are we looking to others to solve their problems for us. Rather, we are wrestling with problems firsthand, formulating and reformulating our questions as we gain further insight into their essence. Each possible solution is itself a problem, in the sense that it needs to be investigated to determine what the group did well, what it did poorly, and what additional questions or opportunities the solution gives rise to. Even if no solution is forthcoming, the process is not necessarily a failure. It may lead to a better understanding of the problem. And the lessons learned may turn out to be more valuable than any solution would have been.

Members of an action-learning group learn about the problems we face and the solutions we devise. But we also learn about ourselves and each other. We become more self-reflective practitioners, knowing what we know but also knowing how we learn. We gain a better sense of our own strengths and weaknesses as learners. Because we understand better the situations in which we learn most effectively, we can create those conditions and enhance learning. We are not only learning but also learning to learn. This is the highest and best meaning of the familiar phrase, "life-long learning." No one knows everything we will need to know. Developing our capabilities as learners is positively crucial for the long-term flourishing of our organizations.

With its roots in the military, after-action review provides a model for organizational inquiry that seeks an enhanced understanding of the nature and causes of events. After-action reviews need not be huge, extremely time-consuming endeavors. They can take place on a quarterly or annual basis in the context of a multi-day retreat. They can also occur everyday, requiring only a few minutes. The name implies that this form of inquiry can be used only in retrospect, but in fact it is appropriate at any point in a process or activity, from beginning to end. It is not necessary that the process by completed, but it must have a starting point and an end point, a purpose, and some definable outcome or outcomes by which performance can be appraised.

The underlying purpose of after-action review is to prevent the unnecessary loss of tacit knowledge. Tacit knowledge is what we know but cannot tell. We know how to ride a bike, but we would find it hard to explain in words to someone who had never done it before. After-action review helps us to transform our private, tacit knowledge to group knowledge, so that each group member can learn from the experience. It helps us become aware of what we know, find words to articulate it, share it with one another, and thus achieve sustainable improvement in our performance.

If a group of people who have worked on a project are about to go their separate ways, we should consider keeping them together long enough to discuss what happened and why. What worked and what did not? What factors contributed to success, and which detracted from it? Where did people function well as an integrated unit, and where did communication or cooperation break down? Were criteria for assessing performance well specified, and what light did they shed on the process?

Several steps are involved in an after-action review. First, key participants need to be brought together, and basic guidelines for the process need to be established. If the right people are not at the table or the process is not well organized, considerable time and energy can be wasted. Key ground rules should be observed. The goal is not to understand who made a mistake. In other words, ascribing culpability is not the point of the review. In fact, blame should be avoided because it inhibits knowledge sharing. The discussion should focus on the goals the group was attempting to achieve, not formulating a new mission statement or conducting a strategic planning exercise. It is important that everyone feel free to contribute, trusting that our perspectives will be welcomed.

It is also important to downplay formal hierarchies. If participants think that those above us in the organization will punish us if we speak our mind, the quality of knowledge sharing will suffer. If we look carefully at what we are doing or what we have done, what can we learn that would help us do better in the future? It often helps to designate someone as a facilitator. The facilitator can ensure that all voices are heard, help draw out insights, and prevent the discussion from descending into recriminations.

An essential question concerns objectives. What did we attempt to achieve, and what did we in fact accomplish? Did we begin with a clear goal in mind? If not, is it any wonder that we are dissatisfied with the results? Do we need to revise our objective? Do we need to develop a clearer sense of the results that we want to assess? At what points have we stepped back to appraise our performance, and what revisions to this schedule would we make in the future? A common mistake is to fail to assess performance more than once during the process. If we wait until the work is finished, crucial course corrections are usually much more difficult to make.

There is a natural tendency to focus on what is going poorly, but it is equally important to consider what is going well. One goal of doing so is to avoid creating an atmosphere of gloom and doom, which can prove enervating. It is important for people to feel that our efforts are bearing fruit. This contributes to a sense of efficacy that is vital to future improvements. Moreover, at least some aspects of a project are almost always going well. By inquiring into the underlying reasons for success, we can improve even further. What people and projects are performing well, and what could we do to make them even better?

It is vital that the insights that flow from an after-action review be shared throughout the organization, beyond the confines of the team that conducts the review. Each group need not repeat the mistakes of every other or be forced to reinvent the wheel of success on their own. There are a variety of means of sharing results, including white papers, newsletters, formal presentations, chat rooms, and informal social events. Ideally, the lessons should be stored in some form that is accessible to others in the future, even after the team members have left the scene.

The fact that there are multiple approaches to organizational inquiry suggests that no single approach is perfect. To say that physicians and healthcare leaders must choose only one approach – action science, action learning, or after-action review – would be like asserting that physicians must choose only one discipline – cardiology, pulmonology, gastroenterology, or neurology – and dispense with the others. In medical leadership as in clinical medicine, the best approach is a pluralistic one, which incorporates familiarity with multiple modes of organizational learning and attempts to capitalize on the strengths of each.

Each approach offers helpful insights on creating and sustaining a learning organization. By studying the different forms of organizational inquiry, leaders can cultivate a deeper appreciation of its benefits and develop an approach best suited to our own organization. In some settings, organizational learning may be an entirely foreign concept, while others may require little more than fine tuning to achieve their full learning potential. Before we can envision how we need to change, we must first understand who we are. The key, however, is to be curious, committed to excellence, and above all, to strive to learn continuously.

Yet learning is not automatic, and only academic medical centers and healthcare organizations that make the investments necessary to do it well can achieve their full learning potential. In effect, leaders must not only want to learn but also learn how to learn, and it is here that the models of organizational inquiry stimulate invaluable reflection and discussion. In learning to learn, we enable ourselves to reap a full harvest from what otherwise might have been the largely fallow ground of our own experience. Every healthcare organization makes mistakes, but the best ones really learn from them.

***

If academic medical centers and healthcare organizations are to thrive in the years to come, it is vital that leaders understand and promote the professional fulfillment of physicians. What makes physicians feel excited about our work and motivated to do a good job? What discourages us, leaves us feeling burnt out, and perhaps even leads us to seek other career options? These are not trivial questions. When work is challenging, promotes our personal growth, and enables us to make an important difference in the lives of others, great rewards flow to the organizations of which we are part, as well as to the patients, students, and communities we serve. On the other hand, if we experience confusion, stagnation, or a lack of appreciation, we are unlikely to perform at our best, and those who depend on us may suffer.

This discussion explores the sources of professional fulfillment among physicians. The term most frequently employed in the literature to describe career contentment is satisfaction. However, fulfillment better captures the sense of professional engagement and reward we need to get at. Satisfaction, from the Latin *satis*, merely means "enough," while fulfillment, from Old English, implies completion, the thorough realization of our potential. Of course, work is not the only factor in the equation of human fulfillment. Personal factors also play a major role. No matter what level of professional success physicians enjoy, we are unlikely to feel fulfilled if our personal lives are in shambles.

Professional fulfillment among physicians has been linked to a multitude of desirable social and financial outcomes. It enhances patients' perception of the quality of healthcare. It lowers turnover, and thereby prevents conditions for others from deteriorating. It helps to lower the rate of health problems among physicians. Physicians' sense of professional fulfillment is positively correlated with patients' adherence to medication, exercise, and diet regimens. Reductions in physician satisfaction are associated with decreased patient adherence to prescribed disease prevention and treatment regimens.

Over the years, many healthcare organizations have attempted to transform uncommitted workers into highly motivated ones. Unfortunately, many efforts, from financial incentives to sensitivity training, have left employers shaking their heads, with no significant increase in employee motivation, satisfaction, or productivity. Why? One possibility is that we have been approaching professional fulfillment from the wrong point of view. Most people tend to view fulfillment and dissatisfaction as two poles of a continuum. For instance, we tend to assume that low compensation causes dissatisfaction, while high compensation promotes fulfillment.

Landmark investigations performed by Frederick Herzberg and colleagues contradict this view. In 1966, Herzberg studied 203 accountants and engineers, hoping to determine what factors contributed to or detracted from their levels of work motivation. He asked two simple questions. First, "Think of a time when you felt especially good about your job. Why did you feel that way?" Second, "Think of a time when you felt especially bad about your job. Why did you feel that way?"

Herzberg found that in addressing each of these questions, respondents did not refer to the same factors. Instead different factors were associated with high levels and low levels of fulfillment. Herzberg called the factors mentioned in response to the dissatisfaction question de-motivators. Interestingly, these tended to be factors extrinsic to the nature of the work itself, including administrative policies, supervision, salary, interpersonal relations, and workplace conditions. The factors cited in response to the fulfillment question he called motivators, and these were generally features intrinsic to work. These included the nature of the work, achievement, recognition, responsibility, and growth.

Herzberg's findings have been supported by numerous studies in quite different populations and work environments, including professional women, agricultural administrators, managers nearing retirement, hospital maintenance personnel, manufacturing supervisors, nurses, food handlers, military officers, scientists, housekeepers, teachers, technicians, women working on assembly lines, and Finnish foremen, among others. Herzberg found that the intrinsically motivating factors challenged people to work more efficiently at a higher level of quality and enhanced fulfillment. If these were lacking, however, dissatisfaction tended not to increase very much. By contrast, the extrinsic, de-motivating factors played the opposite role. When these features were lacking, deep dissatisfaction resulted. However, enhancing extrinsic factors such as compensation and workplace conditions did little to boost performance or a sense of fulfillment.

Herzberg likens efforts to enhance extrinsic factors to recharging an employee's batteries, while enhancing intrinsic factors is like installing a generator in an employee. The former strategy may initially produce benefits, but the ante will need to be raised again and again to maintain the same level of performance. The strategy of focusing on intrinsic factors, by contrast, tends to be self-sustaining, enabling us to become our own sources of motivation. Installing a generator, or attending to intrinsic factors, is the only way to ensure long-term and potentially permanent improvements in performance and fulfillment.

When leaders use extrinsic factors such as salary bonuses and new offices to incentivize improved performance, the extrinsic incentives tend to shift our attention away from the inherently fulfilling aspects of work. As a result, we feel less internal dedication to excellence. We begin to depend on the extra income, and if it is ever removed, or further raises are ever withheld, it seems to be a punishment rather than a mere return to baseline. According to Herzberg, no amount of attention to extrinsic factors will enhance our professional fulfillment or performance beyond the average. In order to achieve greater enhancements, we must focus on the intrinsically rewarding aspects of work.

Herzberg's approach provides the foundation of a strategy for fostering physician motivation and fulfillment. First, we need to identify those positions and aspects of work where changes would not be too costly, attitudes are poor, the costs of de-motivation are becoming high, and increased motivation and fulfillment would make a substantial difference. Certainly, these features apply to many facets of academic medicine and health-care. Second, we need to understand and accept that changes in the nature of our work may need to be made. Often leaders do not immediately recognize that the content of work and the style with which it is performed can or should be changed. Fortunately, the rapidly evolving nature of contemporary medicine has accustomed physicians to change. Third, we need to brainstorm a list of alternative approaches to enriching work. Herzberg recommends that we do so initially without regard to practicality, cost, or time. Later, we can return to the list and weed out ideas that are too costly or impractical. Fourth, we need to screen out suggestions that focus on extrinsic, de-motivating factors, such as financial bonuses.

Another approach to be avoided is what Herzberg calls horizontal loading. Horizontal loading differs from vertical loading in the manner by which the requirements of work are increased. With horizontal loading, relatively meaningless aspects of a job are augmented, resulting in a decreased personal contribution and fewer opportunities for growth in relation to work. Examples of horizontal loading include increasing production requirements, adding fruitless tasks, rotating job assignments, or removing the most challenging portions of the job. The math in all of these examples starts with zero and then multiplies by, adds, or subtracts another zero. The result, of course, is still zero.

By contrast, vertical loading involves increasing the intrinsically motivating features of work, such as responsibility, recognition, and achievement. Examples of vertical loading include increased personal accountability, additional authority, fruitful new tasks, and encouragement to develop expertise in a certain area. Unlike horizontal loading, the end result of vertical loading can be enhanced fulfillment.

Once we finalize our list of options for enhancing the intrinsically motivating features of work, Herzberg suggests that we start implementing them in a small, experimental group. The purpose of utilizing an experimental group is to assess changes in performance, motivation, and sense of fulfillment. Pre- and post-intervention evaluations should be conducted. In order to avoid confounding effects, extrinsic, de-motivating factors should remain unchanged. It is important to anticipate drops in performance and fulfillment during the first few weeks of an intervention, as people acclimate to the new system.

Administrators may find it especially difficult to adjust to the new system due to anxieties about short-term declines in performance. We may also feel as though some interventions are undermining their responsibilities. Over time, however, the rise in physician motivation and fulfillment will be accompanied by a concurrent increase in productivity and quality. With anxieties allayed, administrators may find that we have more time to attend to core managerial and supervisory functions, thus enhancing our own performance and sense of fulfillment.

Because the specific sources of physician fulfillment vary widely among groups of physicians and practice settings, a universally applicable master list of interventions is impossible to compile. The first priority in every case, however, is to accentuate the intrinsically rewarding aspects of the work. Above all, we need to feel that we have made a real difference in the lives of others. As medicine has become more compartmentalized, there is a danger that this source of deep fulfillment is becoming less apparent. For example, reducing face-to-face contact between physicians and patients weakens our relationship and with it physicians' sense that we are making a real difference. To increase the fulfillment of academic physicians, we need to ensure that the intrinsically fulfilling aspects of the work are accentuated, not undermined.

Other fundamental factors related to physician fulfillment are growth and recognition. Given the length and rigors of medical education, as well as the vital role of life-long learning, there is little doubt that physicians must be committed to ongoing intellectual growth. In focusing on the acquisition of knowledge and skills, however, we must not neglect personal and professional growth. Physicians should be encouraged to become involved with organizations and service opportunities that expand our personal and professional horizons. Voluntary service is not necessarily a detriment to efficiency and productivity.

Leaders ignore the subject of physician fulfillment at our peril. For academic medicine and the entire healthcare system to thrive in the coming years, we need to attend more carefully than ever to the factors that enhance and detract from the quality of work we do. If we operate with a clear understanding of the psychology of professional fulfillment and the various organizational strategies that foster it, we can promote a powerful sense of fulfillment among physicians. This, in turn can help to rekindle the noble aspirations that drew us to careers in medicine in the first place.

***

How we get paid can exert a profound influence on what we do. Hence, it is vital that healthcare leaders give some thought to incentive and reward systems. If the goals of the organization and the incentives offered to workers are not aligned, one or the other is likely to suffer. On the other hand, tinkering with compensation is not risk free. Reengineering a compensation system in an effort to manipulate the behavior of highly educated professionals such as physicians is fraught with peril. Over the past few years, some healthcare organizations have moved toward a revenue-based compensation system that introduces a tighter connection between clinical revenue generation and compensation, rewarding people who generate more revenue. Such compensation systems deserve close scrutiny, particularly from an academic perspective.

Proponents of paying health professionals according to the clinical revenue we generate cite several rationales. First, if the people generating the most revenue are not compensated for it, we may grow dissatisfied. Second, providing the same compensation to people whose levels of production are very different can provoke a sense of injustice. Third, if people know that we will be compensated the same even if we generate less clinical revenue, our productivity will tend to decline over time. Finally, giving people a financial incentive to generate more revenue can lead us to work even harder, improving the financial bottom line for both the organization and its employees. Proponents of revenue-based compensation ask the following question: What kind of world would we inhabit if everyone were paid the same, regardless the quantity or quality of work we did?

Yet leaders need to ask ourselves some important questions. The first concerns the relationship between work effort and revenue. Is there sound evidence that the people who generate the most revenue also work the hardest? In many cases, the answer to this question is very much in doubt. A general pediatrician and a neuroradiologist may work similar hours with similar levels of intensity yet generate very different amounts of revenue. Physicians working in settings with poor payer mixes or lower collection rates may generate less revenue, even though we are working as hard as colleagues in other settings. And there is the problem of quality. Practices that maximize revenue may undermine quality of care, by forcing physicians to work faster than we should.

Another question concerns the problem of supporting non-clinical activities. If clinical revenue is the basis for calculating compensation, what will happen to non-clinical activities such as education, research, and service? In terms of the long-term healthcare needs of the nation, a compensation system that precipitates an abandonment of these academic missions would be disastrous. Yet if non-clinical academic missions are to be taken into account, compensation cannot be strictly revenue-based. Teaching medical students does not generate as much revenue as performing medical procedures. To address such concerns, it would be necessary to develop a more inclusive system of assessing productivity that incorporates measures of performance other than revenue. Yet how could we quantify teaching in a way that rendered parameters such as student contact hours and quality of teaching commensurable? How could research productivity be measured: presentations, publications, grant dollars? How could each member's service contribution be measured? It is vital that those who will live with the answers to such questions participate in the development of the system.

A new level of complexity emerges in attempting to capture such diverse variables as clinical revenue, educational activity, research activity, and service activity in a single compensation system. How many student contact hours or peer-reviewed publications is an appendectomy worth? Multiple points of view may be involved in such calculations. At the departmental level, an emergency department may represent a poor source of clinical revenue, and investing more money in emergency services may appear a misallocation of resources. Yet from the medical center's point of view, the emergency department may be a vital component of a larger and financially important service line that includes neurosurgery and cardiology. Moreover, an emergency department physician who contributes relatively little to a department's bottom line in terms of clinical revenue may nevertheless make superb contributions in medical student and resident teaching, or through departmental administration.

A third question concerns the time frame in which compensation systems operate. What will be the longer-term effect of a decision taken to increase short-term clinical revenue? Physicians could probably get more work done and generate more clinical revenue if we reduced the amount of time we spent in face-to-face conversation with patients and families. In the short term, a hospital might benefit financially from a policy of minimizing such conversations. In the long term, however, such interactions may be vital in building patient–physician relationships, generating word-of-mouth referrals, and enhancing physician fulfillment.

A fourth question: what is the role of compensation in motivating and satisfying physicians? Is money the only thing we really care about? If not, where does money rank as a source of motivation, as compared to others such as the opportunity to enrich the lives of patients, the ability to keep growing and developing personally and professionally, the opportunity to sustain a high quality of life outside of work, the level of camaraderie in the workplace, the fairness with which people are treated, the opportunity to play a role in organizational decision making, and our sense that we are excelling at our jobs. Simply paying people more will not necessarily change the quality or quantity of work we do, and cutting pay is no guarantee that people will change the way we work.

There are two major pitfalls in drawing more attention to extrinsic rewards such as pay, which is exactly what a revenue-based compensation system tends to do. For one thing, people may begin to "game" the system, doing things that increase our compensation but do not contribute to the larger ends of the organization. For example, physicians may begin to "cherry pick" work that most increases compensation, and shun work that generates little revenue. Second, focusing on extrinsic rewards distracts us from the intrinsic rewards of work itself. If extrinsic rewards such as compensation supplant intrinsic rewards, then physicians cease to be medical professionals and become mere moneymakers.

The less intrinsically interesting, challenging, and rewarding we make our work, the more important it becomes to bait people to do it through extrinsic rewards. The more intriguing and challenging it is, and the more opportunity it provides for professional discernment and personal growth, the more dangerous it becomes to attempt to manipulate professional behavior through extrinsic rewards. Is medicine an intrinsically rewarding field or not? Should physicians counsel premedical students to consider entering the field only if income is their principal concern, or would we point to other aspects of medicine that make it rewarding? The enthusiasm for revenue-based compensation systems encourages academic leaders to do things to our faculty, rather than working with them. Such systems tend to accentuate differences in power, creating distance and competitiveness within an organization, rather than fostering cooperation and a sense of team spirit. If leaders really want to improve the quality of work our organizations do, we should look for ways to help our colleagues become better physicians.

There is no question that unfair compensation systems represent a real threat to healthcare organizations. Few situations can erode satisfaction and loyalty more quickly. Yet, tinkering with the compensation system is usually neither the most effective nor the safest way of improving a organization's performance. Good people care about more than money, and the amount of money we make is not what we care most about. If some degree of revenue-based compensation is unavoidable, leaders should consider basing it at the level of the section, the department, or the school, and not strictly at the level of the individual. Otherwise, individuals may find themselves increasingly pitted against one another, and the organization to which they belong may disintegrate. It is vital that leaders prevent clinical revenue from overwhelming the other things physicians need to care about.

***

Medicine's leaders need to appreciate the extent to which its future hinges on the quality of research we promote. If the field stagnates for lack of time, funding, or interest, then the development of new and more effective means of promoting health and preventing, diagnosing, and treating disease will suffer. Huge challenges lie before us, including cardiovascular diseases, cancer, dementia, and trauma. To cease to progress is to fall further and further behind. By contrast, playing a leadership role in research is one of the best ways to promote the welfare of patients and ensure productive and fulfilling careers for ourselves and our colleagues. It is vital that future leaders sustain and augment medicine's investigative commitment.

Yet, merely providing more funding for research or granting more academic time to physician–scholars will not get the job done. Research is not simply the product of the amount of time or funding we allocate to it. The best research requires something more, something that speaks to a deeper aspiration in the human psyche. Research represents the expression of a profound desire to know, one of the most characteristic features of human beings. At our best, we investigate things not because someone is paying us to do so but because we want to know. We need to deepen our understanding of this deep desire. The better we understand the nature of curiosity, the better equipped we will be to design careers, departments, and disciplines that give us the opportunity fully to engage this passion.

Why do we seek to know? The question itself manifests the phenomenon it seeks to account for. At one level, to state that human beings desire understanding is simply a matter of definition. This insight provides the opening sentence of Aristotle's "First Philosophy," the *Metaphysics*. To know is what we are naturally inclined to do, just as birds are inclined to fly and fish to swim. Yet the problem goes deeper than this. At times, our desire to know springs from a desire for something else. For example, we may investigate pain in order to prevent or treat it. Among the other ends that inspire the search for knowledge are wealth, power, and pleasure. In each case, knowledge represents a means for pursuing something else.

It is certainly possible to earn a living through the sweat of our brow, but few would dispute that understanding generally offers a less taxing and more effective path to wealth. We can break our backs digging ditches or invent a piece of heavy machinery that can do much of the work for us. The drafters of the US Constitution recognized the power of wealth as a motive when they codified the right to intellectual property in the form of patents (Fig. 3.1). As a means of spurring innovation, individuals receive, for limited periods of time, exclusive license to develop and sell new technologies. The prospect of earning a living, or even getting rich, can act as a powerful inducement to innovation. On the other hand, material wealth has its limitations. As Wordsworth warned,

> The world is too much with us, late and soon;
> Getting and spending we lay waste our powers.

Simply put, the human organism has powers that far exceed acquiring and disposing of money. A life devoted solely to money represents a stunted form of existence.

What good would billions of dollars do a person stranded alone on a desert island? It is not money, but what we can do with it, that makes it enticing. Moreover, there is a limit to how much wealth we can enjoy. Beyond a certain point – a million

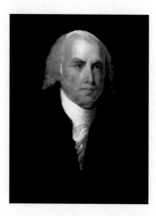

Fig. 3.1 James Madison (1749–1852), fourth President of the United States and principal author of the US Constitution, which sought to promote discovery and invention by codifying a right to intellectual property. The US's is the world's oldest federal constitution, and Madison is widely credited with introducing its tripartite model of legislative, executive, and judicial branches

dollars, ten million dollars, one hundred million dollars – acquiring and spending additional wealth offers little. Besides, some of the most important things in life cannot be purchased at any price. Consider understanding and love. Money allows us to pay our tuition bills, but money alone does not make us any wiser. Trying to buy love merely reveal how poorly we understand it. Finally, a person can try to become wealthy for the wrong reasons or by the wrong means. Consider someone who resorts to criminal activity. Good people recognize that such a person is letting the tail wag the dog.

Power, too, is a problematic justification for the pursuit of knowledge. Power simply means the ability to get someone else to do our bidding. How can we be sure that they should wish to carry out our wishes? Like money, power can be used for good or ill. Some people use power to exploit others, while others use it to enrich lives. There is no guarantee that the exercise of power will redound to anyone's benefit, even the person who wields it. History is replete with examples of individuals who acquired power but then destroyed themselves. And power's destructive potential is not confined to the economic or political spheres. Many powerful people, including Roman Emperors such as Caligula and Nero, were destroyed morally, as well. In the words of Lord Acton, power tends to corrupt, and absolute power corrupts absolutely.

Is pleasure the motive behind research? Is the investigator scratching a mental itch, the itch of curiosity? If so, then our passion for understanding would amount to little more than a dog's desire to fill its empty belly. The scientific mission concerns more than merely pleasing ourselves. The pleasure we take in seeing and hearing things is a sign that knowing is natural to us, but it does not indicate that we seek to know only because it is pleasing. Mere pleasure seekers have not really made their pleasures their own. They are simply following the lead of their instincts. In such cases, the experience of pleasure is a largely passive one, something we could get from a pill. By contrast, the excitement and joy of discovery are active pleasures that arise from the pursuit of understanding.

To understand the true joy of discovery, which differs sharply from mere pleasure, we must first gain a deeper understanding of its meaning. One essential aspect of discovery is the fact that it brings us closer to the world around us. Galvani observed that frogs' legs his wife had suspended by copper wires from the kitchen ceiling were twitching. His curiosity piqued, he went on to demonstrate that nerves conduct electricity and that electrical stimulation plays an important role in muscle contraction. A related principle of discovery is the value of lingering at intersections. Alexander Fleming's first hint of the existence of penicillin came when he observed a lack of bacterial growth in moldy areas of Petri dishes. Instead of discarding the dishes as contaminated, Fleming pursued the matter further, recognizing that "contamination" was giving him the opportunity to study the intersection of two hitherto separated phenomena. Contamination made the discovery possible, in the sense that it could never occur in a perfectly pure, dust-free environment.

Sometimes we need to step outside our comfort zones. Consider benzene. Chemists struggled for years trying to figure out its molecular structure, knowing that it is composed of six atoms each of carbon and hydrogen. X-ray diffraction studies had demonstrated that all of the bonds in the molecule were of the same length, yet each bond was shorter than a single bond and longer than a double bond. How could such a molecule exist? One evening chemist Friedrich Kekule dozed off before his fireplace and began to dream. In his dream, he saw a snake eating its own tail. Suddenly it flashed into his mind that benzene's structure could be that of a ring, in which electrons where "shared" between different atomic bonds through a process he called "delocalization," now known as "aromaticity." At work here is Einstein's famous principle that we cannot solve important problems using the same kind of thinking that defined them in the first place.

When we reflect on these three basic principles of discovery – looking around, lingering at intersections, and stepping outside – we see more clearly that desires for wealth, power, and pleasure are insufficient to account for our desire to know. Beyond each of these desires is the capacity for a far deeper and more engaging experience; namely, the capacity for joy. Joy is born not in repose but in action. It represents more than a mere lightening of the mood. It is a soaring of the spirit. Joy arises in communion with reality itself. It results from knowing not merely what happened but how it happened and why. As we understand more deeply the how and why of events, we also gain a deeper insight into what is taking place. We understand more deeply what each thing is, and how it came to be.

This is the fundamental genius behind the co-called allegory of the cave in Plato's Republic (Fig. 3.2). We are like people living underground, watching the shadows of figures projected onto a wall by the light of a fire behind us. Should we arise and explore the cave, we could see the objects themselves and the fire that illuminates them. Should we explore still further, we might even find our way out of the cave, and come to stand in the sunlight. Initially, the bright light of day would blind us, but eventually our eyes would adjust and we would be able to see things as they really are. Plato suggests that we have the ability to see beyond ourselves and the superficial appearances of

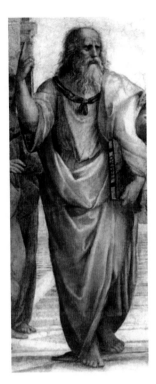

Fig. 3.2 Detail from Raphael's *School of Athens* depicts Plato (428–348 BC), bearing a copy of his *Timaeus* in one hand, his other hand pointing heavenward toward the realm of higher things. Alfred North Whitehead once declared that "The safest general characterization about the European philosophical tradition is that it consists of a series of footnotes to Plato"

things. Our minds are capable of traveling to distant times and places, including celestial objects on the other side of the universe, whose light as been traveling toward us for billions of years.

As our understanding reaches out and connects us with the world and its inhabitants, we begin to experience true joy. It is above all through understanding that we fulfill our nature as knowers. Aristotle thought that in discovering the world around us we also bring it more fully into being. Other entities, from tiny bacteria to massive stars, are unable to know themselves and the world to the same extent as we. Our understanding penetrates cellular metabolism and nuclear fission in ways that are utterly impossible for bacteria and stars. In this respect, human beings play a vital role in the universal scheme of things. We do not merely exist as the kinds of creatures we are but we also help to realize the natures of other things. In studying them, we bring to light aspects of their being they themselves cannot elucidate or wonder at.

Knowing is the distinctively human activity, and it is in knowing above all that we complete ourselves and the world around us. We seem to have been constructed to know, and the world around us seems to have been constructed to be knowable. In doing science, we help to fulfill both our own natures and the natures of the things we know. A flower may be able to spawn another flower, but it does not know what a flower is or what a flower does. Though we never become something other than what we are, we can know their essences, and in so doing complete both their nature and our own. It is in exercising this almost divine capacity that we participate in reality's most sublime joys. Discovery is important not only for the sake of other things but above all for itself.

Chapter 4
Styles of Leadership

Metaphors powerfully shape our lives. Consider, for example, the metaphor of war. A declaration of war between two sovereign states signals that each intends to defeat the other, perhaps even to destroy the other's capacity to wage war. During the Vietnam era, the President of the United States declared war on some quite different sorts of foes, poverty, and cancer. In these cases, the use of the term "war" was largely metaphorical. Neither poverty nor cancer has an army and both are impossible to locate on a map. We can pinpoint geographical areas where the rates of poverty and cancer are high, but we cannot pinpoint opposing troops or their commanders. Yet by declaring "war" on poverty and cancer, we predisposed ourselves to see them as definable foes, as enemies that could be vanquished, and as causes around which a nation could rally.

Metaphors are also at work in our professional lives. They shape a leader's sense of mission, the strategies by which we pursue our goals, the resources we take to be at hand, and the styles in which we interact with colleagues. Consider, for example, the role of a department chair. There are a number of different metaphors that we may employ, consciously or unconsciously, in thinking about what a chair should be and do. We might, for example, liken the chair of an academic medical department to a firefighter, policeman, cheerleader, manager, hero, or coach. By exploring such metaphors in light of our own expectations for chairs, we can arrive at a more realistic and fruitful image of what chairs do.

R.B. Gunderman, *Leadership in Healthcare*,
DOI 10.1007/978-1-84800-943-1_4,
© Springer-Verlag London Limited 2009

At a time when many medical departments have difficulty filling leadership positions and the people who assume the roles find them more and more difficult to play, examining our image of the chair is especially important. This discussion explores one of these images in depth—that of the chair as firefighter. In this model, the leader's job is to patrol the organization putting our fires. Such fires include budgetary shortfalls, personality conflicts, perceived inequities, lapses in service, and hosts of other problems that beset most departments on an at least occasional basis.

In many settings, such problems are routinely dumped on the desk of the chair. When referring health professionals have difficulty getting a consultation scheduled in a timely fashion, we call the chair. When staff members feel we are being overworked or underpaid, we call the chair. In many departments, such fires erupt not sequentially, but concurrently, with multiple burning at once. The chair is frequently pulled simultaneously in multiple different directions. When people sense that the chair is not focused on our particular complaint, we attempt to turn up the heat to ensure that our concern moves higher on the chair's priority list.

A chair who closely resembles a firefighter is in trouble. For one thing, this approach places the chair in a purely reactive mode, responding rather than planning, and carrying out rearguard defensive actions rather than creating opportunities. Instead of helping to develop an agenda for the department, the chair allows it to be controlled by others, including people who may not have the best interests of the department at heart. As soon as one problem is solved, others appear to take its place. For chairs who dislike strategy or perform poorly as planners, the firefighter mode can be a comfortable one. With many crises looming on the radar screen, there is no opportunity to put away the fire suit and axe and begin thinking about what the department should strive to become.

The image of firefighter transforms the chair into a creature of crisis management. To spend each day putting out fires can be rewarding. You feel needed because people keep coming to you to point out the blazes they expect you to put out.

Grappling with crises can be exhilarating. Some chairs may experience a kind of adrenaline rush. Yet over time, the crisis mentality begins to take a toll on the chair's energy level and sense of well being. It also interferes with planning. Merely preventing the buggy whip factory from burning down is not good enough when the age of the automobile is dawning. Medical practices and healthcare organizations need to do more than react to the initiatives of others. We need to play an active role in shaping our own future.

Some leaders who never manage to extricate themselves from the firefighter mentality adopt a defensive strategy. They use the crises they face as a shield with which to defend themselves. When someone presents with a problem, they simply say that they cannot handle it at present because they are totally occupied putting out other fires. Yet, there is no guarantee that the first fires that come to the chair's attention are the most important ones. The people who shout the loudest do not necessarily have the most to say. Over time people may cease to share important information. They may feel that the chair is too busy to listen to them or that their voice will never be heard over the din of others.

A major problem with firefighting is captured in this nostrum: The squeaky wheel gets the oil. In such an environment, there is a natural tendency for the number of complaints to escalate. Why? People soon realize that the chair devotes most of his or her time to problem solving. The only ticket of admission to the chair's attention is a problem, and the bigger the problem, the better. The more important you judge yourself and your constituency to be, the more problems you bring to the chair.

Fires do not always arise spontaneously. Some are set. Colleagues feel incentivized to light fires beneath the chair to make things happen. Some people decide that the best strategy to increase their compensation is to threaten to quit. Yet acceding to such demands lands the chair in a dangerous whirlpool. Once one group's demands are met, another group determines that they too need a raise. They announce their intention to seek employment elsewhere. The frequency and intensity of blazes spirals upward.

Another problem with fighting fires is a lack of continuity of purpose. People need to know what the organization and its leader stand for. They need to know what counts most in the leader's mind. They need a clear understanding of the organization's mission, as well as the future people are called to promote. Leaders who spend all day trying to put out fires soon discover that they contribute little to the organization's momentum. Their divergent vectors cancel each other out, adding up to zero. Leaders find themselves expending considerable energy but accomplishing nothing. People in the department suffer for lack of a clear sense of direction.

Many problems that draw chairs into an increasingly reactive mode can be delegated to other people with fewer strategic responsibilities. For example, a vice chair of clinical operations, ideally someone who enjoys face-to-face interaction and monitoring day-to-day operations, can be empowered to address routine clinical problems. The chair needs to know what is happening, but need not assume responsibility for personally addressing every concern.

Another problem with firefighters is the fact that they are not architects or builders. Except for safety considerations, we do not expect them to help us construct homes, office buildings, or community centers. We look to them to keep buildings standing. Firefighters are caretakers who maintain the status quo. They strive to return to baseline, a quiet state in which nothing is burning. There are, however, circumstances in which a fire can be a good thing. Sometimes we benefit from creative destruction. Cities such as Chicago and London are more beautiful, functional, and safer because a good deal of rickety old, haphazard construction was cleared by a great fire. There are situations in which creative destruction is precisely what is called for. We need people in our departments who are not afraid of change, and who recognize that creativity and improvement are impossible without it. A chair committed to making the department better needs a vision of what better means and a willingness to make the changes necessary to achieve it.

When we reflect on what a leader needs to be, the image of a firefighter should not be the first one that comes to mind.

Chairs cannot ignore clouds of smoke when they appear, but they need not be the first to attack every single blaze. Colleagues who help chairs avoid this fate, enabling them to focus most of their energy on creating opportunities, are providing a vital service, and contributing as leaders in our own right.

***

Recent commentators have argued that conventional measures of intelligence such as intelligence quotient (IQ) explain only part of achievement. Empirical research into the connection between IQ and overall success has shown that many people with high IQs are not particularly successful, and many people whose IQs are not particularly high do very well. In his book, *Emotional Intelligence*, Daniel Goleman argues that much of the variance in performance can be explained in terms of non-cognitive, "emotional" abilities. These include self-awareness, the management of moods, self-motivation, empathy, and the management of relationships. Some critics have objected to calling such abilities "emotional intelligence," in part because they are not strictly "emotional" in nature. Others point out that such abilities are not fixed and innate in the same way that psychologists usually understand "intelligence." Nevertheless, the general idea of emotional intelligence offers insights from which many leaders can benefit.

As formulated by Goleman, the first component of emotional intelligence is self-awareness. Whether we are playing a sport or diagnosing disease, it is vital that we monitor our reactions to the people and events around us. We need to recognize when we are feeling enthused and when we are feeling disheartened. If we do not attend to these reactions, we will have difficulty differentiating between the times we should persist in what we are doing and those when we should try something different. It is important to be able to name our emotional states because people who can do so generally exhibit a more sophisticated and nuanced self-awareness than those who cannot. For example, can we distinguish the embarrassment we might feel at failing to detect an important finding on physical examination from the indignation we would experience if colleagues went out of their way to point out the mistake to others? If all we can say for such states is that we are feeling "down," then our depth of emotional self-awareness is poor, and our effectiveness is likely to suffer.

To enhance performance in this area, Goleman suggests that we conduct an emotional self-inventory. Am I quick to grow frustrated and lash out at others, or someone who never loses my cool? Do I grow discouraged easily, or do I tend to forge ahead despite repeated disappointments? Am I a loner, to whom colleagues do not tend to form attachments, or am I everyone's best friend? The key objective of an emotional inventory is to recognize our strengths and weaknesses and look for ways to augment or compensate for them. If I have a short fuse, I might seek out approaches to avoid blowing my top.

A second component of emotional intelligence is managing moods. There is some value in simply monitoring how we feel, but if we are to perform at our best, we also need to be able to influence it. People can be intellectually brilliant, but so poor at coping with frustration or disappointment that we could never succeed. Encountering disappointment and frustration, emotionally intelligent people do not fly off the handle. We are able to hold such reactions in check, remaining focused on the task at hand. By contrast, emotionally immature people are ruled by passions and lose focus in trying circumstances.

The goal of managing moods is not to squelch all emotion. Emotion provides the wind in our psychological sails. People who flourish are not passionless automatons. We care about what we do. Striving hard to ensure that a research project bears fruit, or that students get a good education, or that patients receive first-rate medical care is very important, and no one in their right mind would recruit a truly apathetic physician. However, we need to ensure that expressing our passion does not undermine the very things we are passionate about.

Managing moods does not pertain solely to negative emotions such as anger, jealousy, and fear. It is equally important for positive emotions, such as compassion. If we are going to provide the best care for patients, we need genuinely to care about them. When a physician, nurse, or technologist genuinely cares about a patient, it shows through in our interactions with them in countless ways. We could try to develop detailed rules for what to say and avoid saying, but such rules become largely superfluous if patients see that they matter to us as human beings. By cultivating our compassion, we become more effective health professionals.

A third component of emotional intelligence is self-motivation. People who perform at a high level tend to be very self-motivated. We have a relatively clear sense of what we are trying to achieve, and our desire to reach our goals is strong. It would be difficult to convince us that they were barking up the wrong tree or that our aspirations were unimportant. Moreover, we do not rely heavily on encouragement from others. There is a fire burning in our belly that enables us to persist despite setbacks or discouraging words from others.

In a time of relatively rapid change, it is especially important that healthcare organizations find leaders with strong internal compasses. When the external environment is shifting, it is easy to get sidetracked and start moving in the wrong direction. Good leaders are able to keep our gaze fixed on the larger goals the organization needs to pursue. We are sufficiently passionate about them that external events do not throw us off course. Key figures in the history of medicine, such as Vesalius and Harvey, were so focused on objectives that they never gave up, even though others regarded their projects as quixotic (Fig. 4.1).

What motivates us as physicians? What are we really trying to achieve? What would it mean if our principal mission were to augment incomes? Would this be a goal we could get truly excited about? What would it mean to the future of our field? Alternatively, what if our passion were to make the biggest possible contribution to the health and well-being of patients? Is this a goal we could get excited about? What would such a motivation portend for the future of our field? It is not enough to be merely pig-headed. To be truly effective, we must also operate from the right motives.

A fourth component of emotional intelligence is empathy. Physicians are not just machines for grinding diagnoses out of large collections of facts. Some people are "book smart" but "people challenged." Each of us knows someone who is highly

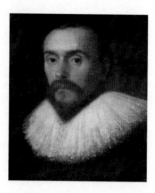

Fig. 4.1 William Harvey (1578–1657), who conclusively demonstrated the circulation of the blood in man and animals. A master rhetorician as well as experimentalist, Harvey ranks as perhaps the most influential English-speaking physician in history

intelligent in conventional terms, the smartest or most knowledgeable person in the room, yet whose effectiveness is limited. When it comes to selecting candidates for admission to medical school, we must look beyond fund of knowledge and IQ and to emotional intelligence. We need to select for and cultivate empathy.

Effective leaders not only recognize how we are feeling but also actually care about us, as well. They convey such genuine concern by listening attentively to what we have to say and attending to our non-verbal signals. Electronic means of communication such as telephone and email are, emotionally speaking, relatively impoverished. As a result, empathetic leaders strive to communicate face to face, which enables them to attend to the full range of interaction. When we sense such genuine empathy in a leader, it inspires trust and loyalty.

As leaders, do we care about our colleagues? Do we take an interest in their personal lives? Do we know when they get married, or have children, or suffer a loss? Or do we remain so aloof that we are always the last to learn of such events? To be sure, there is a difference between being empathetic and prying into others' lives, and it is important to respect privacy.

Yet it is even more important that we convey to others how important they are to us. They need to know that we are willing, even eager to offer comfort and support should the need arise.

The fifth and final component of emotional intelligence is managing relationships. It is naïve to think that successful leaders simply see where our organizations need to go and then tell others what to do in order to get there. People who have never been in uniform often suppose that the military works this way – that commanders simply bark out orders and subordinates blindly submit. In fact, however, good leaders need to develop the respect and loyalty of the people we work with. Simply seeing what needs to be done is not enough. We also need to cultivate strong relationships.

Why do people show up at work everyday? If it is merely to collect a paycheck, then the organization is in trouble. Few of us could afford to keep working if we were not paid, but this does not mean that we do it for the money. In the best of all possible worlds, we come to work because our patients, our colleagues, and our organizations really matter to us. We are passionate about what we do. And we recognize that we could not do it without the people we work with. They are part of us, and we are part of them, and together we are capable of promoting important missions that we could not achieve independently.

All discomfort is not necessarily bad, just as all comfort is not necessarily good. Comfort can lead to complacency and obsolescence. Discomfort can spur creativity and risk taking. Managing relationships means knowing when tension can be good for the organization and when it is likely to prove counterproductive. To tell what level of comfort is appropriate, we need to communicate. Communication enables us to learn as individuals, as teams, and as organizations. It also helps to forge a vibrant sense of collegiality and shared identity.

When we select students for admission to medical school and postgraduate training programs, we need to look at least as carefully for emotional intelligence as for intellectual intelligence. Scores on standardized tests are often less important than self-awareness, self-motivation, and empathy. I have known learners whose academic records were mediocre, but who identified a keen interest in some aspect of medicine, recognized what they needed to do to pursue it, and proceeded to achieve great things. Their IQs were not especially high, but they were able to draw upon their high emotional intelligence and eventually outperformed others with greater cognitive ability.

To what resources can leaders turn to develop our emotional intelligence? One of the deepest sources of insight into the variety of forms of emotional experience is imaginative literature. At it best, it affords nearly unparalleled glimpses into what it means to be human, enabling us to cultivate our emotional sensitivity and providing powerful portraits of the consequences of both poorly and highly developed emotional intelligence. While the dramas of Shakespeare and the novels of Tolstoy and Dickens immediately recommend themselves, one of emotion's most accessible and penetrating observers is Jane Austen, whose Sense and Sensibility, Pride and Prejudice, and Persuasion represent masterpieces in this regard (Fig. 4.2).

***

In contemporary academic medicine, diversity is a misunderstood topic. On the one hand, proponents of affirmative

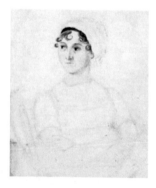

Fig. 4.2 Jane Austen (1775–1817), whose *Sense and Sensibility*, *Pride and Prejudice*, and *Persuasion* are among British literature's most penetrating depictions of the richness of emotional and social life

action in admissions and hiring argue that sexual, racial, and ethnic preferences are necessary to remedy past injustices and achieve a more balanced and representative student body. Opponents counter that merit is the only just basis for selecting one candidate over another, claiming that any system of preferences only perpetuates discrimination. The debate extends beyond admissions to faculty hiring and promotion policies and even to decisions about how to invest endowment funds.

What is the proper role of diversity in our medical schools and healthcare centers? Before we can answer this question, we need to examine some more basic ones. What is diversity? What happens to an organization or a community when diversity is lacking? What does diversity offer in the way of benefits? Should leaders in medicine strive to promote diversity throughout our organizations? If diversity is worth pursuing, what can we do to promote it?

We can distinguish between at least two dimensions of diversity. First, there are fixed dimensions of diversity. These include attributes over which we have no control, such as age, sex, skin color, and innate abilities. The other dimension is open. It is made up of elements that are at least partly subject to choice, including educational background, marital status, religious beliefs, and work experience. As we increase diversity in a system, we move from simplicity to complexity and from the monotonous to the polyphonic.

What happens to an organization or a community when diversity is lacking? A lack of diversity can breed both ignorance and complacency. As Socrates (Fig. 4.3) repeatedly argued, the last people to embark on a search for understanding are those who believe they already know everything. He regarded the presumption of omniscience as the worst form of ignorance. At the levels of the individual and the organization, ignorance and complacency rank among the most important barriers to discovery and innovation.

Such intellectual blinders may be self-imposed or externally imposed. When self-imposed, we take our narrow horizons for granted, believing that things could not be otherwise. We suppose that ours is the only valid point of view and tend to regard

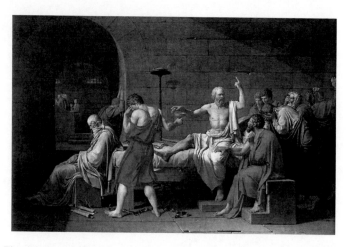

Fig. 4.3 David's *The Death of Socrates* (1787), depicting the great philosopher drinking Hemlock and willingly submitting to the death sentence
pronounced by a jury of 500 of his fellow Athenians. Though Socrates
(469–399 BC) left no writings, he remains one of the most influential
thinkers in world history

engaging others in conversation as a waste of time. When the
blinders are externally imposed, they represent a form of tota-
litarianism. In the extreme, this is the sort of thought control,
terrifyingly envisioned by C.S. Lewis in *The Abolition of Man*
and George Orwell in *1984*, that threatens to undo conscience.
If we are forbidden to think differently, we never reexamine our
assumptions or feel the need to explain ourselves, and this
arrests our moral growth and development.

Consider the impact of diversity in the history of human
cultures. The genius of the ancient Athenians sprang in part
from their sea-faring economy, which put them in constant
contact with other peoples who worshipped and acted differently. At the opening of Plato's Republic, Socrates is just
returning from the Piraeus, the Athenian port and site of out-
landish religious festivals. This contact with other cultures sets
the stage for his penetrating inquiry into the nature of piety and

justice. The moral bounty of diversity can be immense. Only when we realize that our way of thinking and doing is not the sole option can we examine our own way of life and gain true insight into others. To paraphrase John Stuart Mill, those who view their own way as the only way do not understand even that.

During the Western medieval era, China represented perhaps the most advanced civilization on earth. But then it turned inward, isolating itself from contact with other cultures and becoming increasingly ossified. Totalitarian regimes such as the former Soviet Union were doomed not only by their dilapidated economic systems but also by their success at suppressing diversity of thought, which undermined innovation.

In the world of biology, diversity is a vital ingredient in a recipe for a robust and resilient habitat. A wide variety of species is a sign of a thriving ecosystem, while ailing environments are characterized by monotony. Genetically speaking, inbreeding fosters biological brittleness, while diverse systems are much better equipped to adapt and rebound from stresses.

Human communities are likewise enriched by diversity. Groups composed of a diverse membership enjoy a competitive advantage over homogeneous ones. They bring more points of view to the table. The very activity of working together, recognizing and appreciating the distinctive contributions of different perspectives, helps build a sense of community. It encourages respect and mutual understanding. Former US President Jimmy Carter once suggested that the most appropriate image of our nation is not a melting pot out of which we pour a single alloy, but a rich mosaic made up of many diverse elements, each of which remains true to itself. So long as the differences between us do not incite destructive conflicts, our communities are strengthened.

Conventional aspects of diversity such as race and gender are very important. Yet leaders cannot afford to ignore another type of diversity that often tends to get overlooked – intellectual diversity. We need to continue to promote equality of opportunity in the fixed dimensions of diversity, but we also need to attend to its open, voluntary aspects, including diversity among the disciplines. We need to seek not mere tolerance or peaceful coexistence, but rich dialogue. Communication and sharing of knowledge are key. What are our colleagues in other disciplines working on? What are our students learning in their classrooms, clinics, and laboratories? How can interaction with people outside our own organizations enrich our work?

If we want our students and colleagues to realize their full potential, it is vital that we nurture their ability to look at questions from multiple points of view. Homogeneity pacifies us and puts us to sleep, while diversity prods us, stretches us, and invites us to reexamine and reformulate what matters most to us. We need to welcome not only dull harmony but also dynamic tension. If our interactions fail to make us uneasy, then we are probably not trying hard enough. This renders a relish for spirited dialogue a crucial leadership attribute. Consider the classroom. Instead of rewarding students for merely memorizing answers, we need to encourage them to explore questions. The best students should set their sights not on imitating the faculty but on challenging and surpassing us. The same goes for our colleagues and future leaders.

Recombination and mutation are the engines of intellectual creativity. Our classrooms and our board rooms need porous walls. We need to foster the intercourse of diverse perspectives. By deeply understanding diversity, we can uncover many opportunities to combine and recombine ideas and life experiences and promote new forms of hybrid vigor.

There are numerous practical steps we can take to promote diversity, the appropriateness of which will vary from institution to institution. Examples in the academic setting include encouraging faculty members to team teach interdisciplinary courses, teaching introductory courses outside our disciplines, recruiting faculty with interdisciplinary scholarly interests, enabling learners to choose or even create interdisciplinary courses of study, developing course assignments that challenge learners to integrate learning from two or more disciplines, and holding regular interdisciplinary colloquia featuring outside speakers.

A medical school composed of castles and fiefdoms is not an intellectually fertile environment. We cannot achieve true diversity merely by arranging different disciplines or intellectual points of view side by side. To achieve genuine diversity, different perspectives need to become engaged with one another in meaningful dialogue. Castles and fiefdoms are not only less interesting but also less secure. We should regard the boundaries between us not as invisible fences that we dare not transgress, but as frontiers that beckon us to mutual exploration. It is not by isolating ourselves but by interweaving ourselves that each of us becomes a truly distinctive yet integral thread in the tapestry of academic medicine.

For future leaders in medical and healthcare, intellectual diversity is not an option but a necessity. This means that we need liberally educated leaders. To be liberally educated is to be free. A liberal education is one that prepares us to make our own informed judgments and to choose freely for ourselves. We are no longer slaves to the past, simply parroting what we have been told. Our deepened understanding and compassion prepare us to give of ourselves for the benefit of others, the excellence of character we call liberality. Diversity is essential to liberal education. It nurtures intellectual and moral discernment, helps us situate our organization's challenges and opportunities in the context of a wider world, and prepares us to lead responsible lives not only as leaders but also as human beings and citizens.

***

When colleagues choose to switch from full-time to part-time employment, or express interest in retiring at an early age, they may be warning us that their work experience is not what they expected or hoped for. Leaders who understand the ingredients that go into improving work can take steps to improve both our own lives and those of our colleagues, enabling everyone to come to work each day with a deepened sense of dedication, camaraderie, and fulfillment. Because work is such a substantial part of our day, successful efforts to enhance work can dramatically enrich quality of life. Such improvements can benefit not only health professionals but also the patients we serve.

Work improvement has been a subject of sporadic study for decades, but a volume on the subject by a team of psychologists,

Howard Gardner, Mihalyi Csikszentmihalyi, and William Damon has clarified the key ingredients of good work and the strategies leaders can employ to promote them throughout their organizations. "Good work" can mean at least two things: (1) the quality of our experience at work and the contribution work makes to our overall quality of life and (2) the quality of the product or service we deliver. The two concepts are clearly related because people who are proud of their work are more likely to enjoy it, and people who enjoy what we do are more likely to do a good job. Because the two are so frequently intertwined, this discussion will not draw a sharp distinction between them.

Gardner and colleagues criticize recent studies of the work experience that have employed reductive or atomistic methods. These largely confine themselves to breaking down complex work performances into their elementary components. In health care, total quality management (TQM) and continuous quality improvement (CQI) sometimes exemplify this approach. Applying such methods to medical practice, we have been able to measure how long it takes to produce a particular product, such as a complete physical examination of the respiratory system. By analyzing the complex chain of steps involved in production, we have developed strategies by which to reduce costs, increase throughput, and improve error rates. These are laudable goals, and the quality movement has achieved important successes that have allowed physicians and other health professionals to work more efficiently and do better work. However, such quantitative methods frequently overlook the quality of our work life.

In order to explore quality of work life, we need to ask some additional questions: Why do we do the work we do? What do we want from our work? What could be done to help us make the most of our work experience? Most of us do feel better about our work when sources of inefficiency and error are reduced, but few of us assess our overall satisfaction strictly in terms of productivity. Electronic health information systems are helping to improve work satisfaction by reducing lost information, eliminating physical exertion, and increasing productivity, but technological approaches alone cannot address all aspects of work. Before we focus on the quantitative and technological aspects of work improvement, we must first understand in qualitative terms how physicians and our coworkers understand the quality of our work experience.

We must be willing to look beyond throughput and error rates to address three larger questions. As formulated by Gardner and colleagues, the first of these questions is this: How do we assess what we do at work in the context of the wider world? We need to see our work as making a contribution to life beyond our organization. If workers believe that the world would not suffer were our organization simply to disappear, then dissatisfaction and burnout are likely. No matter how quickly we produce a product, we are unlikely to feel good about the work we do if that product does not make the world a better place.

Leaders should ensure that people who work in our organizations enjoy ample opportunity to see the difference the organization makes in the lives of patients it serves. Systematic approaches to assessing quality of care that focus on outcomes can be helpful because they encourage every member of the department to think about how work helps reduce costs or improves patient comfort, functional status, or longevity. On a more personal level, leaders need to foster the development of a culture that cares about work experiences, where people share with one another accounts of what a job well done has meant to a patient or family. A department that insulates us from the opportunity to see the larger meaning of work is asking for trouble.

A second crucial question is this: how do we know when someone is doing a good job? If the only indicators of job performance we attend to are throughput and error rates, then we are courting dissatisfaction. For example, suppose departmental receptionists are evaluated based strictly on the speed with which they field calls, and physicians are assessed strictly in terms of the number of patients they see. These are seriously impoverished indicators of work quality because they leave out a number of vital quality indicators. Do the people whose calls the receptionists have fielded feel that their questions were answered promptly, courteously, and correctly? Did the physicians do a good job of diagnosing and prescribing treatments for their patients' ailments?

We need to expand our conception of good work to encompass not only speed and accuracy but also relevance, helpfulness, and an overall sense that we are performing at our best. Having someone with a stop watch looking over your shoulder all day can prove counterproductive if it does not respect the broader meaning of good work in the minds of the people doing it. When we feel proud of the work we are doing, we find work itself more fulfilling. Leaders need to look for ways to help physicians, nurses, business managers, receptionists, and other employees perform at our best. We often understand our work and the factors that contribute to quality better than anyone. Getting us actively involved in assessing and improving quality not only improves performance but also proves rewarding in its own right because we feel more of a sense of ownership in the work we do.

A third vital question concerns how we become good at our work. If we adopt as our definition of improving work minimizing the number of errors that occur at each step in a work process, then leaders may begin to regard the people who perform those steps as cogs in a machine. This is a surefire way to de-motivate the best workers, who regard ourselves not as interchangeable parts, but as unique and committed professionals, on whose distinctive efforts the mission of the organization depends. Leaders should strive to create a culture in which the organization invests in workers, by helping us further our education, encouraging us to emulate people we admire, and becoming personally involved in serving as role models for others.

By posing these questions, leaders can diagnose and treat organizational disorders that compromise the quality of work. If the members of a medical group feel that we are losing autonomy, the ability to control the structure and quality of our work, then our sense of commitment to work is likely to suffer. Likewise, if we feel that we are being manipulated into increasing throughput at the expense of quality, many of us will begin to seek opportunities elsewhere. Suppose, for example, that throughput could be increased by insulating proceduralists from all contact with referring physicians, making it possible to spend every minute performing and never fielding other physicians' questions or learning more about patients. On the surface, this might seem a beneficial change in workflow, leading to improved "productivity." In the long run, however, it would likely undermine continuing education, compromise the relevance and quality of consultation, and make it harder for the physicians in question to appreciate the value of contributions to referring physicians and patients.

Where should leaders who want to improve the quality of work focus our attention? Gardner and colleagues recommend focusing on what they call the three M's: mission, models, and mirror. The mission of an organization is the answer to the question, what are you trying to achieve, and how does it serve others? If we do not know the answer to this question, we cannot perform at our best. Given the chance to discuss the mission, many of us feel both grateful and reinvigorated because it helps us to see more clearly the target we are trying to reach. Each of us truly wants to make a difference.

Even senior people in a field may lose sight of the mission from time to time. In general, this is most likely to occur in situations where we are overworked, where substantial changes are taking place in the work environment, or when we feel we have little or no autonomy in defining, assessing, or improving our work. In a medical practice that is losing personnel at a high rate, an attitude of survivalism may quickly predominate. People begin to see the organization as a sinking ship from which we should extract as much as possible before it goes under. We may start basing decisions on our own short-term financial or career interests, rather than the long-term mission of the organization. We may lose interest in efforts to improve quality of work life, build infrastructure, or enhance patient care. To get such an organization back on track, leaders need to refocus attention on the mission of the organization and each person's role in achieving it.

The second M is models. We need to interact with others we regard as worthy of emulation. Principles and techniques are important, but until we see them put into practice by real people, they often remain too abstract to bring to life. Role models are absolutely vital to an organization, putting a human face on the ideals the organization is pursuing.

In the case of the disintegrating practice, an effective leader would need to find individuals in the organization that people admire and draw attention to their attitudes and work practices. The goal should be to get people focused on a shared vision of excellence, rather than picking the organization apart based on pet peeves and vested interests. Regular meetings of the group would be vital, so that people could discuss their personal visions of what a good department should be doing. Individuals from other practices that have surmounted similar challenges in the past could be recruited to participate in such meetings, sharing their experiences and recommendations. What were the key factors that turned their practice around? How did key role models help people focus on the longer-term missions of the organization? What pitfalls would they recommend avoiding? It is good to discuss theories of work quality with management consultants, but there is no substitute for face-to-face discussion with peers who have faced the same problems.

The third M is mirror. We need to step back and examine the direction we are taking, the people and organization we are becoming. When people look in the mirror, we need to ask ourselves, "Are we proud of what we see here? Would we be willing to hold ourselves out as a model of how this work ought to be done?" Many organizations end up looking quite different from what they intended simply because we never took the time to look at ourselves in the mirror.

There is an important difference between making a living and making a life. In reflecting on the quality of our work life, it is vital that we address these questions: What do the many hours we spend each week at work contribute to our larger sense of what we want to do with our lives? How do they enrich the lives of others? What can we do to make work more enriching for everyone involved? If we really care about the work we do, not merely because we collect a paycheck, but because we see the difference it makes in the lives of others, then the quality of work will improve. Such an improvement will benefit not only physicians but the people physicians work with, and most importantly, the patients for whom medicine exists in the first place.

Chapter 5
Hazards of Leadership

Being a leader means dealing with complaints. When people perceive a problem, we naturally seek out someone in authority to share it with, and leaders need to think carefully about how to respond to such interactions. There are times when complaints seem the bane of our existence. It can be both disruptive and frustrating when the smooth flow of a day is interrupted by a phone call, email, or visit from an unhappy person. When this happens, we need to bear in mind that frustration may have been building up over a long period of time. By the time it finally bursts forth, it may burn like steam jetting from a ruptured pipe. The sting is heightened when complaints seem personal, even though the leader bears no personal responsibility for the problem.

Some people never learn how to complain effectively. They suppose that, in order to be taken seriously, their complaints must be couched in terms of catastrophe, coercion, and threats of retribution. Their favorite word is "unacceptable," and they frequently send copies of every complaint to the most senior people in the organization, even before the responsible person has been notified and given a chance to respond. Every expression of concern is accompanied by warnings that if the situation is not rectified "immediately," they will be forced to refer all of their patients to another facility, seek employment elsewhere, and so on. Such attitudes are unfortunate, and one thing leaders can do to amend them is to excel at handling complaints.

R.B. Gunderman, *Leadership in Healthcare*,
DOI 10.1007/978-1-84800-943-1_5,
© Springer-Verlag London Limited 2009

The word "complain" comes from the Latin com- (with) and plangere (to strike or beat the head or breast as a sign of grief). At one time it denoted the expression of sadness or regret, as in bemoaning. During the twentieth century, particularly in business circles, it has acquired the connotation of finding fault. Several decades ago, the corporate functions now designated as customer service and service recovery were housed in the complaint department. Today, when people complain, they are not merely finding fault, but expressing annoyance, and even leveling an accusation.

From an enlightened leader's point of view, complaints should not be seen as threats. Embedded within most complaints is an opportunity – at times a very important opportunity. Chicago department store magnate Marshall Field once said,

> Those who enter to buy, support me. Those who come to flatter, please me. Those who complain, teach me how I may please others so that more will come. Only those hurt me who are displeased but do not complain. They refuse me permission to correct my errors and thus improve my service.

In other words, complaints can be one of the most important sources of constructive feedback for an organization. They point out things that the organization is doing wrong and reveal opportunities to do things better.

If we can weather the stormy exterior of many complaints, we can discover a silver lining within. To reap its rewards in improved performance and morale, however, we need to adopt several leadership habits. First, we must make ourselves and the organization open to suggestion, actively soliciting advice from those we serve. It is important to resist the temptation to insulate ourselves from bad news. Second, we need to develop means of sharing complaints with everyone who stands to benefit from them, ensuring that valuable learning opportunities are not squandered. Many complaints are not received by the people who most need to hear them. Third, we need to create a culture that shares complaints without fear of giving offense. Shooting the messenger accomplishes nothing.

To protect against these dangers, healthcare organizations need to develop systems for handling complaints and educate members in using them effectively. Fortunately, other industries have been working on this challenge for many years, and healthcare leaders need not reinvent the wheel. The number of options is great, but one system worthy of consideration is the so-called LEARN approach. Practiced by major corporations such as the Marriott group, LEARN is an acronym whose letters stand for Listen, Empathize, Apologize, React, and Notify. Behind LEARN is the idea that every person in an organization who receives a complaint or suggestion should ensure that each of these five steps are taken.

Listen – Listening to complaints sounds easy, but it can be very frustrating. Many of us tend to cut off the complainant at the first opportunity. Such reactions might be justified in terms of efficiency ("I know what he is unhappy about, so let's start working on fixing it"). From the complainant's point of view, however, simply being listened to is a key factor in satisfaction. Moreover, some complainants need some time to think through their concerns while they speak, and they may take a minute or two to get around to what really concerns them. Individuals who feel our blood pressure rising as we listen should keep reminding ourselves that the complainant is usually trying to give us something of value; namely, a free user's assessment of the organization's performance.

Empathize – Empathy means seeing others' concerns from their point of view. One of the greatest hazards in any service industry is the failure to appreciate the customer's perspective. In medicine, patients and colleagues are the analogues of customers. When they lodge complaints, they are telling us what our service means to them. The same may be said for complaints arising from the staff of the organization. Leaders need to know what our colleagues care about and seek to understand their point of view. So long as it is sincere, telling someone that we understand how they feel, or that we can understand how frustrating a situation must be, can establish a rapport that facilitates finding a remedy. If we truly do not care about the people we serve, then an empathetic attitude will be difficult to project. But what would this say about our status as a caring profession, or a healthcare organization's prospects for survival?

Apologize – An apology need not be an admission of fault. If patients complain because they were kept waiting longer than they expected, a physician can apologize without taking personal responsibility. In some cases, the delay may have been the result of unforeseeable and uncontrollable events, such as an unexpected medical emergency. Yet the person lodging the complaint is not responsible for such an emergency, and a simple explanation of what happened, followed by an expression of regret, can be a powerful anger solvent. If the complaint stems from a foreseeable and preventable failure, then an apology is even more important. Few experiences undermine trust as much as an attempt to withhold or hide information that a reasonable person would want to know. A sincere apology goes a long way toward assuring the aggrieved that we have dealt with them openly.

React – Listening, empathizing, and apologizing are vital, but they are not enough. If the organization merely hears complaints but does nothing about them, a vital opportunity has been lost. Reacting effectively to complaints means actually doing something about them. In some cases, adverse situations can be addressed by a single person or a small group of people. For example, a complaint that staff members are not introducing themselves to patients can be rectified by speaking directly with those concerned. Other complaints require a wider response. In order to define the individual or organizational opportunity a complaint represents, we may need to discuss it with others, particularly specialists in service recovery. In every case, however, the goal is not merely to get this irate person off our back, but to learn from the experience and avoid similar problems in the future.

Notify – The notification step is especially important in learning organizations where frontline employees are empowered to address complaints as they arise. From a customer's point of view, such a system is superior to one that requires complainants to put their concerns in writing and wait weeks for a response. The danger of immediate response systems, however, is their tendency to hinder wider awareness of each complaint, thus depriving others of a valuable learning opportunity. Leaders need to put in place systems that ensure that the appropriate person is notified each time a complaint is registered. We need to provide opportunities to share best practices about how complaints have been addressed.

An organizational culture that does not learn from complaints is likely to find itself increasingly out of step with the people it serves, particularly in a period of relatively rapid change. To keep improving, we must keep learning, and to keep learning, we must keep listening. Complaints are never as pleasant as compliments, but they are usually more instructive and almost always more frequent. The key is to learn to regard them not as personal attacks but as learning opportunities.

***

The situation is familiar to any physician who has faithfully attended sessions during a large professional meeting, attempted to read every page of the month's journals, or simply spent an entire day at a museum. Before long, we reach a state that cognitive psychologists have sometimes called "information overload," a term coined in 1971 by futurist Alvin Toffler. Information overload is a state in which we are confronted with so many inputs that our cognition becomes dulled, decision making impaired, and mental exhaustion sets in. This state threatens our ability to perform effectively, particularly for leaders who have many constituencies competing for our attention. In order to cope effectively with information overload, we must first understand it.

Technological change is increasingly outpacing biological change. We are developing exponentially more and more effective and efficient ways to collect, store, and disseminate information. By contrast, the amount of information we are capable of assimilating is changing rather slowly, if at all. Merely reveling in our ability to encounter more and more information would be as sensible as gloating over our ability to load more weight on our bodies. At some point, it starts slowing us down, and eventually it may break us.

We can claim that new information technologies are at our service. We may even console ourselves with the notion that we can slow down the flow of information whenever we wish. In fact, however, we often more closely resemble slaves of the new information technology than its masters. Increased access to information brings something to our lives, but it consumes something else. In the words of Herbert Simon, "It consumes the attention of its recipients. Hence a wealth of information creates a poverty of attention, and a need to allocate that attention efficiently among an overabundance of information sources that might consume it." Instead of necessarily liberating us from the workplace, information technology also turns out to be a Trojan horse that allows work to invade our personal lives.

More information is not necessarily better information. In some cases, seeing more fails to enhance our performance, and may actually degrade it. Increasing the frequency of updates from monthly to weekly, from weekly to daily, from daily to hourly, and from hourly to by the minute will not necessarily prove beneficial. How frequently do we really need to check our email? The habit of seeking more information can paralyze us in situations where we know enough to make a decision and further delay may cause damage.

The information age is a boon to our well-being only if we make good choices about which sorts of information to access. Merely enlarging the library does no good, if we find ourselves overwhelmed and less capable than ever before of discerning which books and journals to read. Being able to store more and more data and to manipulate those data in an ever more sophisticated fashion is of little value unless it enables us to do better work and lead better lives. To cope with the information avalanche, we need to pay more attention to the kinds of information we have available. We need to make some informed choices about what we attend to. In operating an automobile, we do not focus all our attention on the surface of the road. Professionally speaking, what do we really need to know to lead effectively, and what can we afford to disregard?

We need to recall the concept of the signal-to-noise ratio. Consider a chest radiograph. The signal in such an image is carried by the information-bearing photons striking our retinas. By contrast, photons from the sun or overhead lights constitute noise because they bear no diagnostic information.

They only make our pupils contract and drown out the signal on which we need to be focused. In order to improve the signal-to-noise ratio, we can do one of two things. First, we can increase the signal. In a lecture setting, this might involve amplifying the voice of the presenter. Alternatively, we can decrease the noise, by keeping side conversations to a minimum. Determining the best approach to the signal-to-noise problem depends on the particular situation at hand.

Taking anything to the limit is usually a bad idea. If we turn up the gain on a computer monitor excessively, we are presented with a screen full of static. If we turn it down too low, we face a blank screen. To respond appropriately to the challenges of information overload, we need to keep in mind what we are ultimately hoping to accomplish. A more aesthetically pleasing image is not always a more diagnostic one. As the cost of disseminating information has fallen, the cost of receiving information has increased. The signal-to-noise ratio is always at risk. This accounts in part for the recent resurgence of interest in meditation and prayer. We feel a greater need than ever before to exit the information superhighway, take time out, breathe deeply, and experience the sound of silence. Often it is only in silence that we hear the call of the truly important.

What do we really need to perform at our best? Where does doing our job begin to infringe on our personal lives, ultimately undercutting our professional effectiveness? There is a difference between knowing everything and being knowledgeable. The annals of neurology furnish examples of remarkable individuals with prodigious memories, known as mnemonists. They are capably of easily memorize reams of information, such as listings in a telephone directory. However, such people may suffer, precisely because they cannot distinguish the signal from the noise.

The problem of information overload imposes responsibilities on our professional organizations. It is great to share, but there is a limit to how much information each colleague wants and needs. The leader's job is to help colleagues appreciate the wealth of information that is available, but responsibility for accessing most of this information should reside with each person. Rather than "push" everything we have available, we need to allow colleagues the opportunity to "pull" from a menu what they want to see.

People in leadership positions often suffer most from information overload. The chair of a department or president of an organization may receive dozens or even hundreds of emails each day. Colleagues may reflexively copy superiors on each piece of correspondence, forgetting that several dozen others are doing the same thing. To be knowledgeable means not only having a lot of information at our fingertips but also distinguishing between the less relevant and what we really need to know. A true expert is not the person who knows the answer to every question but the person who knows what questions to ask. The best physician is not a walking data repository but a good investigator who knows what to look for. Even a photographic memory does not make a person wise. The information age makes it more vital than ever before that we cultivate our ability to discern and focus on what is really most worth knowing.

***

Why do health professionals fail in leadership positions? One reason is a lack of education in management and leadership. Consider a hypothetical newly installed chair of an academic department. This leader graduated at the top of his class in medical school, performed brilliantly in residency, and advanced rapidly through the academic ranks, having been awarded a number of large extramural research grants and published dozens of papers in refereed journals. However, this same high-achieving academic physician has never taken a single course in management or leadership and has little knowledge or experience in key leadership competencies such as communication, organization, and financial management. His expertise as a physician vastly outweighs his expertise as a leader, and this leadership deficit compromises his chances of success as chair.

What can leaders and prospective leaders do to avoid this pitfall? One approach is to acquire formal training in leadership. Formal coursework is available through colleges and universities, and organizations such as the American College of Physician Executives offer additional leadership courses specifically tailored to physicians. Numerous commercial organizations also offer opportunities, and some professional organizations have recently developed leadership programs. The most important objective of such programs is not to supply participants with an academic degree or professional certification, but to enable them to develop knowledge and skills integral to successful leadership.

An underrated priority in medicine is developing leaders before we assume key leadership positions. Too many physicians recognize the need to cultivate our leadership expertise only after we become chair or dean, by which point it may be too late. We should educate for leadership at every phase of medical careers, beginning in medical school and residency. Because many aspects of leadership cannot be conveyed through books or lectures, physicians at every stage of development need to pursue service opportunities that test and refine our leadership capabilities. Current leaders should recognize that one of the most important contributions of a good leader is the development of colleagues for leadership. Truly great leaders promote the leadership potential of those around them.

Another major pitfall is the failure to adapt. Different departments and schools have different cultures, and a person who functions effectively in one may perform poorly at another. To a substantial degree, success hinges on recruitment, finding the best candidates for the organization's needs. There is much that prospective leaders can do to buttress our chances for success. We need to ask ourselves some questions: What is the culture of this organization? What kind of leadership are people accustomed to? What challenges and opportunities require the greatest focus? After exploring these and similar questions, prospective leaders should then consider whether we are well matched to the organization's needs. An organization in crisis may need a strongly authoritative hand, but most departments will benefit more from a collaborative approach.

Effective leaders do not set out on day 1 bending everyone to their own will. They are usually consensus builders. In some cases, they may be able to rely on their native brilliance and sheer force of will, but consensus building usually requires listening and learning. Listening helps leaders know what others think, and it gives people the sense that our leader values the people in the organization. When the mandate for change is strong, the period of time available for acculturation may be brief. The better informed and more widely appreciated a leader's plans for an organization, the better the prospects for success. Likewise, the greater the number of people who believe we have played an important role in developing the strategic plan, the greater our commitment to it. Great leaders devote just as much time and effort to building personal loyalty as formal authority.

The demands on a leader's attention are many. Successful department chairs must attend to intradepartmental matters, interdepartmental matters, and relationships between the department and the hospital, other healthcare organizations, healthcare payers, vendors, and the community at large. Some leaders experience other demands on time and attention, such as service in local, state, and national organizations. Many academic leaders also continue to devote a portion of time to clinical practice. In some cases, these other concerns can prove positively overwhelming, diverting so much energy away from leadership responsibilities that the organization begins to suffer. Leaders should regularly consider whether extra-departmental activities consume too much time. At the very least, leaders should be upfront about commitments, and regularly listen to colleagues to determine if they have concerns in this area.

If leaders have a clear grasp of the "to do" list, it is not difficult to determine if important decisions are being made and important projects are being delivered in a timely fashion. In many cases, leaders can increase effectiveness by collaborating and delegating more effectively. It does not make sense for leaders to spend large amounts of time doing things that someone else in the organization could do at least as effectively and at lower cost. Often it is sufficient simply to know what is happening, and the leader need not be the one making everything happen.

The most egregious leadership pitfall is not incompetence but malfeasance. Numerous technical errors of leadership can be forgiven. A leader can miscalculate staffing requirements, fail to budget appropriately for capital acquisitions, and perform poorly as a public speaker or manager of meetings. But a leader who misappropriates funds, falsifies documents, engages in inappropriate relationships with coworkers, succumbs to substance abuse, repeatedly lies to colleagues, or breaks the law is unlikely to get a second chance. No one is above the law or the ethos of an organization, which leaders should not merely abide by but exemplify. One of the worst things colleagues can do is to ignore such misconduct. There are few more dangerous invitations to misconduct than a personal sense of invulnerability, and no one does a leader any favors by aiding and abetting it.

For many leaders, a strong personal faith and an abiding commitment to family and community provide a strong bulwark against temptation. A good rule of thumb is to ask the question, "Would I be ashamed to tell my spouse, children, or best friend about what I am doing?" If the answer is yes, it suggests that a change of course is probably in order. It is usually helpful to develop a close working relationship with at least a few colleagues who can act as sounding boards and advisors for difficult decisions. Leaders have an opportunity to set high standards of character for an entire organization, enhancing mutual respect and enabling everyone to take more pride in our work.

***

Great leaders are not people who have never known failure. They are people who deal with failure effectively, learning from it in ways that enhance performance. Great leaders are not flawless but resilient. Some of us are more resilient than others, but each of us can take steps to enhance resilience in our organizations. We can not only bounce back from failure but actually learn and grow from it. To do so, we need to understand resilience better, especially its sources in medical practice and health care.

One source of resilience is a sense of collegiality, community, and solidarity. When we feel isolated and alone, our clarity of purpose and level of energy tend to suffer. Interrogators usually try to isolate prisoners for precisely this reason. By contrast, when we believe that others are with us, we draw from a deep wellspring of hope and encouragement. This is why the military goes to such great lengths to develop solidarity and comradeship among soldiers. They know that, under difficult circumstances, a close-knit unit will function much more effectively than one whose members know and care little about one another.

Numerous factors in contemporary medicine tend to undermine this sense of collegiality, taking a toll on the resilience of leaders. One of the most important is competition. All physicians serve the health of our patients and the public. Yet contemporary medicine is characterized by increasing competition. We compete with one another for patients, in part because our livelihoods depend on attracting patients who can choose other providers. This strife can prevent us from sharing our experiences with colleagues, for fear that we would be undermining our competitive advantage. As a result, collegiality and professionalism may suffer.

Competition need not necessarily undermine collegiality. In some cases, physicians who compete directly with one another may become and remain good friends. Competition only undermines collegiality if we see one another as locked in a zero-sum game, where one person's gain requires another's loss. If the size of the pie is fixed, taking two pieces instead of one means someone else must do without. When we believe that there can be no winner unless someone loses, then competition exacts a very high price. Yet there are competitive scenarios in which no one needs to lose. For example, physicians can share stories of errors and setbacks in ways that allow everyone, including speakers as well as listeners, to learn and improve.

As every competitor can win, so every competitor can also lose. A lose–lose situation often arises around the precious resource of time. In some practice environments, being busy, even to the point of working unreasonably hard, has become a badge of pride. Physicians who dare to talk about leisure activities, family life, and community service may be regarded with disdain, even ridiculed. "If you have time to talk about such matters, then you are not busy enough." This ethos erodes resilience in two ways. First, when physicians have no time to talk, we cannot build relationships with colleagues. Second, how can resilience flourish among people who are chronically exhausted and leading one-dimensional lives?

The same can be said for fear vulnerability. Some physicians suppose that revealing any weakness, such as anxiety, fatigue, or ignorance, is a sign of failure. We try to project an image of infallibility and invulnerability. Displays of emotion seem intolerable, and we go to extreme lengths to avoid revealing our feelings. As a result, our ability to learn from our own experience is undercut. We work so hard building walls to protect ourselves and prevent any hint of feeling from showing through that we end up completely isolated from those on whom we depend. We may appear strong, but our isolation actually renders us brittle and subject to burnout.

By what indicators can we assess physician resilience? Productivity and revenue are not good candidates. In the short term, physicians who isolate themselves may be able to sustain deceptively high levels of productivity. To get the work done, we avoid spending any time or energy developing relationships. Yet with time, productivity, recruitment, turnover, and fulfillment all suffer, as does morale.

To promote physician resilience, we need to understand the factors that make the practice of medicine a meaningful and fulfilling calling. One such factor is recognition, an acknowledgment of the value of the work we do. How often do we pause to acknowledge the outstanding work of colleagues? Have we organized our practices so that we see the difference our work makes in the lives of others? If we feel starved for acknowledgment and praise, it becomes more difficult to recognize others. On the other hand, physicians who feel that we are doing a first-rate job will tend to have higher levels of resilience.

There is no surer way to discourage highly educated and dedicated professionals than to deprive us of the opportunity to see the difference we make in others' lives. Treating the practice of medicine like piecework inevitably undermines morale. This does not reflect any character flaw or a defect in the way we select, educate, and promote physicians. Quite the contrary, it reflects a fundamental feature of the human psyche. Whenever we begin organizing and evaluating a relationship-centered calling such as the practice of medicine as though it were an assembly line, we inevitably undercut relationships and sow the seeds of demoralization.

Physician resilience hinges less on productivity and income than on inspiration. We need to see our daily work as part of a larger system of meaning. If inspiration is in short supply, we can look outside medicine to art, poetry, music, and faith. Sometimes we need to recall that suffering is as old as humanity itself and that the effort to relieve it represents one of life's noblest callings. It helps us to see ourselves as part of the extraordinary healing tradition that stretches back through Morgagni, Harvey, and Vesalius to Maimonides, Galen, and Hippocrates (Fig. 5.1). If we organize the practice of medicine appropriately, we discover that one of the greatest sources of inspiration is the patient, in whose life story we are privileged to participate. The patient–physician relationship is not primarily a contractual one. It is not a quid pro quo, but a trust.

Physician resilience is highest if we recognize the close connection between becoming better doctors and becoming better human beings. The excellences of a good physician – courage, respect, and practical wisdom, among others – are also the excellences of a good person. It is impossible to cultivate them solely in the personal or professional sphere without cultivating them in both. To do so, we need to approach each day with curiosity and hopefulness, a love of learning and a conviction that through our efforts we can enrich human life. Such outlooks can manifest themselves everyday through the work we do.

Some health professionals have come to regard the hospital as a hostile environment. We feel that others are constantly looking over our shoulders, trying to catch us making a mistake. We feel that we are being subjected to unreasonable expectations concerning documentation and patient throughput. We feel that "guys in suits" are constantly telling us how to

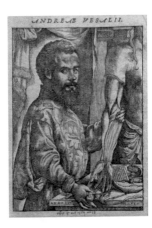

Fig. 5.1 Andreas Vesalius (1514–1564), in a portrait from his monumental 1543 treatise, *On the Workings of the Human Body*, one of the most influential writings in the history of medicine. More loyal to the truth than to tradition, Vesalius did not hesitate to point out errors in the teachings of his great predecessors, Aristotle and Galen

practice medicine. Such perceptions may bear a grain of truth. Yet what we see around us is powerfully colored by what we have inside us. If we know our gifts and enjoy regular opportunities to put them to work, even deep hostility may melt away.

Again the patient can play a crucial role. Do our work routines permit good conversations? Do we get to know patients well enough to appreciate their biographical differences? How often are we learning something important from them, and how often are we putting such lessons to work to help others? One way to create such opportunities is to thank patients when they teach us something, letting them know how we expect to use what we have learned to help someone else, perhaps even someone we have not yet met. By cultivating and expressing such gratitude, we open up new wellsprings of resilience on which we can draw when the going gets tough.

Bad things will never stop happening. Medicine is a matter of life and death, and it will always challenge us deeply, as physicians and leaders. The question is not, "How can we insulate ourselves against all failure and suffering?" but rather "How can we care to the best of our ability?" Resilience is not about imperviousness or impermeability. It does not mean building our fortress walls higher and thicker to keep unpleasantness at bay. Building higher and thicker walls, we eventually discover that what we intended to be a fortress is really a prison. Resilience is about facing up to failure and regret and finding ways to carry on more wisely and compassionately because of them. Far from breaking us down, setbacks give us the opportunity to find a newer and more complete wholeness, and this is exactly what resilience is all about.

Chapter 6
Ineffective Leadership

One of the biggest mistakes a leader can make is to allow a culture of debate to dominate a culture of dialogue. To see what such a shift would look like, we need only turn to our popular culture. When contemporary talk radio and cable news programs feature issues of the day, they increasingly seek out colorful individuals of diametrically opposed points of view. Why? Conflict boosts viewership. In the ratings race, heat trumps light. The participants in such contests often have little interest in promoting a comprehensive or balanced perspective. Instead each attempts to shift the balance of opinion by presenting a radical and uncompromising extreme. In such an environment, civility and good sense suffer, and talking heads tend to morph into shouting heads.

The ascendancy of debate threatens the thoughtfulness that characterizes a learning organization. The word debate is derived from the Old French *debatre*, meaning to fight or contend. Debate implies conflict. Broadcast media did not create it. They have merely magnified it to a new level. What do the combatants seek? Not mutual enlightenment. They seek victory. Where do debaters stand with respect to the truth? Truth is not a matter of complete indifference. After all, exposing the falsity of an opponent's argument can score points. In debate, however, truth represents a mere means to another end: conquest. Should embarrassing facts emerge, the consummate debater can be relied on to ignore, suppress, or "spin" them into irrelevance.

R.B. Gunderman, *Leadership in Healthcare*,
DOI 10.1007/978-1-84800-943-1_6,
© Springer-Verlag London Limited 2009

This rather unflattering contemporary portrait of debate has a forerunner in the culture of the ancient Greeks: the Sophists, whose name means wise. Sophists such as Gorgias were itinerant debate coaches who traveled the region offering lessons in rhetoric. Like contemporary high school debaters, who find out which side of a proposition they will defend by drawing from a hat, the Sophists did not care which side of an issue their pupils were called on to argue. Wisdom was less important than victory. Making the weaker argument appear stronger? Making the stronger argument appear weaker? Not a problem for the Sophists, so long as their side prevailed.

There is a resurgence of the sophistic spirit in professional schools today. Thanks in part to broadcast media, many students now think that discussing an issue means deciding whether you are for or against it and then defending that position to the bitter end. They expect a good argument, and some faculty members, lured by the sirens of "lively discussion" and "energetic student participation," are inclined to give it to them. Debate, however, is not what professional education should be about.

Truly professional education should be about something quite different: dialogue. Dialogue may not generate as much heat as debate, but it generates a good bit more light. Our word dialogue is derived from the ancient Greek *dialogos*, which in turn derives from the roots *dia-*, meaning through, and *logos*, meaning word or reason. A dialogue proceeds by and through words. The parties to a dialogue aim not to defeat one another, but to enlighten one another. It is not a conflict but a shared inquiry. In contrast to the debater's zero-sum game, in which every victory must be accompanied by a loss, dialogue permits both parties to emerge from their discussion enriched. Both can benefit from a shared pursuit of enlightenment.

In ancient Greek culture, the paradigmatic dialogist was Socrates. Socrates possessed all the skills of a master debater. Yet he deployed them not in order to defeat his interlocutors, but to pursue enlightenment. The Socratic Method does not consist of relentless interrogation, badgering and even intimidating students in the manner of *The Paper Chase*'s Professor Kingsfield. The true Socratic Method is not about showing learners or colleagues who is boss. Instead it embodies the realization that true knowledge is born of discovery. Only by treating those who work for us with profound respect can we inspire them as co-investigators.

Socrates was sometimes likened to a stingray. He aimed to produce a state of *aporia*, puzzlement or wonder. He did so, however, not to paralyze but to invigorate. If we suppose we know all the answers, we will never inquire. But if the limitations of our views were brought to light, we might seek better ones. True dialogue is grounded in synergism. Sharing our understandings enables us to gain insights impossible to achieve in solitude. We discover that our preconceptions are not the only options. We learn to look at questions from multiple points of view. By uniting in the pursuit of understanding, we reach cognitive wholes that exceed the sums of our parts.

Such an attitude shines through in genuine conversation, where the goal is not to silence others, but fully to elucidate their points of view. In true dialogue, it is vital that we bring our deepest thoughts and experiences into play. The sharing of such perspectives provides the fertile soil in which discovery and creativity blossom. If wisdom could be transferred from one person to another like water flowing through a straw, Socrates might have been a conventional teacher. Because it cannot, he sought to engage his interlocutors in a dialectical process of shared investigation. He did not encourage memorizing formulae or vetting prejudices. Instead, he would have us examine ourselves, the ideas we care about and the lives we hope to lead.

Socrates was keener on asking questions than supplying answers. His method embodied the understanding that all great discoveries in the sciences and arts spring from skepticism, a readiness to question what we think we know. Money and power meant little to him in comparison to the capacity to inquire. He saw in an uneducated slave as fertile a mind as the most urbane aristocrat. From Socrates' point of view, death is not the worst of fates that can befall a person. Far worse is to become a "misologue," a hater of discourse. We become misologues when we get burned so many times by debate that we stop believing in the possibility of genuine dialogue.

To become open to the possibility of genuine dialogue, we must see ourselves not as passive spectators but as active participants, indispensable partners in the pursuit of wisdom. We need to set aside our prejudices, to push the envelope of our own understanding. The pursuit of wisdom must not be commandeered by the dictates of rhetorical advantage. To remind us of the difference between debate and dialogue is one of the most important missions of contemporary professional education. Learners who emerge from our classrooms confusing the two will be poorly equipped to think clearly, to stimulate genuine conversation, and to share knowledge effectively. They will be ill prepared to flourish as human beings.

What can we do to foster genuine dialogue in contemporary medicine? While the diversity of environments precludes any single formula, here are some questions that are likely to play an important role in a fruitful approach:

> Does every argument have two and only two sides? What do we gain, and what do we give up, by viewing our lives in such terms?
>
> When we win a debate, what do we win? When we lose a debate, what do we lose?
>
> What are the differences between debate and dialogue? How might genuine dialogue open up possibilities for victory by both parties?
>
> How can we promote dialogue in our classrooms and boardrooms?

There is a great deal at stake in the choice between debate and dialogue. Do we wish to create organizations composed of mere debaters who fritter away their energy trying to win zero-sum contests? Or do we wish to produce dialogists, who cultivate conversations from which all participants can emerge enriched? Our leadership style can be one of the best antidotes to a popular culture often dominated by diatribe and indoctrination. It is medicine's best hope for proving that words are not weapons, but windows of discovery.

***

Some academic medical departments are inadvertently undoing ourselves, and in the process pulling down health care with us. In the interests of increasing revenue and reducing costs, we are placing ever increasing clinical workloads on the shoulders of academic physicians. Some years ago academic department chairs began to voice concerns about the amount of academic time traditionally afforded faculty members. In economic terms, this time could be considered a fixed cost from which departments derived little or no marginal revenue. Chairs were asking themselves, "Why should I pay faculty members a full-time salary if they are clinically productive – and by and large, financially advantageous – only 60% or 80% of the time?"

As a result, many academic departments have migrated toward a model that more closely approximates community practice. More faculty members are being paid largely or even exclusively according to our clinical productivity. Those who seek higher levels of compensation are expected to devote more of our time to clinical work, the activity that generates the most revenue. Moreover, periods of time when academic physicians are assigned to clinical duties have become more intense than ever before, leaving less and less energy for non-clinical pursuits. The ability to devote substantial amounts of time to academic work in education, research, and professional service is at risk, and in some cases, undergoing rapid erosion.

Departments that follow such a path may soon discover that they have been penny wise but pound foolish. In the short term, such policies foster solvency, by increasing clinical revenues and reducing costs. Assuming that there is additional clinical work to do, every additional hour that an educator or researcher spends in patient care incrementally boosts the clinical productivity of the faculty. In the short term, it provides a bigger return on the department's investment in faculty salaries. In the long term, however, policies that substantially reduce or eliminate academic time often amount to eating medicine's seed corn. The harvest of that seed, creative thinking and innovation, represents the future of academic medicine and the entire medical profession.

**

In a rapidly changing world where healthcare organizations must innovate to compete effectively, academic medicine's most precious long-term resource is not the clinical productivity of its practitioners. It is our imagination, our capacity to find both better ways of doing things and new and better things to do. A vision of merely generating more clinical revenue and reducing costs is not a truly academic vision. Any academic department devoted solely to such a vision represents a community practice that happens to be situated in an academic medical center. There is nothing ignoble about providing high-quality, cost-effective healthcare services. In fact, this should be a goal of all medical practices, academic as well as community based. However, it is self-contradictory to extol the academic missions of education, research, and service while adopting systems of compensation and reward that focus exclusively on clinical productivity.

Such policies overlook the innovation-promoting policies and practices of many of the world's most successful corporations. Unlike some academic medical departments, top corporations realize that their performance is tied to investments in workers, especially those whose innovations are crucial to the organization. An academic physician I know is fond of likening the practice of medicine to piece work. In his mind, physicians and factory workers both turn out their product one unit at a time, and such productivity is the means by which the organization generates revenue. A department's mission, as he sees it, is to make its faculty as clinically productive as possible, at least up to the point that perceptions of overwork begin to drive workers away. In the ideal, he would like to see physicians scheduled and compensated accordingly.

Likening the clinical operations of an academic department to an assembly line might have seemed apt in the industrial age. But in the information age, when innovation is key to remaining strong, it distorts more than it reveals. Even the twentieth century champion of the assembly line, Henry Ford, was eventually forced to confront the limitations of his model. Once competitors adopted his industrial techniques and began introducing their own innovations, Ford failed to respond. For example, General Motors made automobiles available in colors other than black. Ford's stubborn commitment to the past nearly destroyed his company.

The moment we cease to innovate is the moment we begin to become obsolete. Yet we can only innovate if we have time and energy to do so. How do great companies foster innovation? One of the twentieth century's most innovative corporations, 3 M, developed a policy of permitting its scientists and engineers to devote a portion of their time to projects about which they were passionate. On this discretionary time, usually 15% of their work week, they were free to do what interested them. No supervisor told them what they had to do. From a short-term perspective, such a policy seems ill advised, because it seems to take some of the most highly educated and expensive resources in the company out of the productivity loop. During that time, they seem not to be contributing to the bottom line, at least not as measured by the next quarterly profit/loss statement or annual report.

Yet some of the most important products in 3-M's history grew out of this discretionary time. In the 1920's, one of the company's engineers chose to disobey a direct order to abandon a project to improve the process of painting automobiles. Carrying on with the project on his own time, he developed what came to be known as Scotch masking tape, one of the most successful products in the company's history. From a short-term perspective, he seemed to be wasting time, but from a longer-term perspective, he did far more than any of his supervisors to add value to the company and its customers. This and other examples prompted 3-M's leadership to make discretionary time an organizational policy for its research scientists. Over the years, discretionary time has produced a handsome return on investment.

Companies like 3-M not only encourage their employees to pursue their curiosity but also work hard to ensure that the insights such projects spawn are shared throughout the organization. It is not enough to produce great ideas. It is necessary to share them throughout the organization, so that people learn from one another. At 3-M, employees with discretionary time meet together to discuss their ideas for projects, provide updates, and monitor progress. When this happens, new sparks are ignited, and creative people fan one another's flames. Moreover, the organization is better positioned to take advantage of new insights. If people in medical departments meet regularly to talk with one another and work together as team members, we can devise more effective ways of carrying out our daily work, from scheduling patients, to developing and implementing new technologies, to improving the quality of education and research.

The annals of 3-M furnish another notable example of the value of discretionary time. One researcher at the company was disappointed in a new adhesive he had developed, which seemed not to stick very well. A colleague was annoyed by the fact that pieces of paper he was using as bookmarks in church hymnals kept falling out, making it difficult for choir members to find their place during the service. The second researcher realized that the "defective" adhesive might be a perfect remedy. The two researchers coated pieces of paper with the new adhesive and started using them, first at church and later around home and office. Soon others were requesting their own supply. Thus was born another of 3-M's most profitable products, Post-It Notes. Had the researchers confined their attention to what the company told them to do, the product would never have emerged.

There are other benefits of discretionary time. First, it enhances recruiting. Talented and capable people do not want to spend their lives working for an organization that tells us what to do every minute of the day. We expect to be creatively engaged in our work, to be solving problems, and to be developing new ways of doing things. We want the freedom to grow into our best selves. To a prospective employee, a policy of discretionary time is an important indicator that such creativity is valued by the organization. It shows that the organization recognizes its workers as the engines that make it run, rather than the converse. By contrast, an organization that merely offers more money may have problems that force it to pay more to attract labor.

Discretionary time also promotes both full engagement in work and organizational loyalty. Workers who think our employer is counting on us to help shape the future of the field are much more likely to find and seize new opportunities than workers in organizations who feel we are treated as mere machines for grinding out work. People who are under so much pressure to produce more work that we dare not think about anything else are unlikely to contribute creatively to the organization. And when a better offer comes along, promising either more money or more comfortable working conditions, we are likely to accept it. Because of a lack of intrinsic motivation, such people are more likely to burn out and retire sooner. It is easy to recognize when we are in the midst of such an organization because people never get together to talk about their ideas.

Innovation takes time – specifically, time to talk and time to think. If the time to think is squeezed out of academic medicine, then innovation is going to be squeezed out, as well. If a department expects its faculty members to tend to their teaching, research, and service responsibilities on our own time, it sends the implicit but unmistakable message that such activities are viewed as hardly worth paying for. No matter how much lip service such an organization pays to innovation, we are going to feel that we are being penalized for doing it. On the other hand, if a department does a good job of encouraging faculty members to spend time on non-clinical pursuits and holds faculty members accountable for results over the long term, then performance is likely to improve. Such an approach enables faculty members to incorporate new perspectives into our clinical work and to bring lessons from clinical work to other academic activities.

Given the huge benefits of innovation, it is unsurprising to learn that Internet giant Google encourages its software engineers to devote 20% of their time to work-related projects they are passionate about and 10% of their time to anything they care to work on. It is surprising, however, to learn that Google does not restrict this policy to engineers. In fact, its discretionary time policy applies not only to engineers but also to all of its employees. In other words, the organization takes seriously the creative potential of every one of its workers. As expected, this makes it relatively easy for Google to attract and

retain top talent. When Google interviews prospective
employees, the discretionary time policy is one of the first
things they ask about.

From a short-term perspective, discretionary time may seem a
misallocation of resources. If the goal is merely to improve productivity and revenue in the next quarter, then increasing the
proportion of time that physicians spend on clinical work may
seem the prudent policy. In fact, we can boost the bottom line even
higher by simply reducing the number of physicians. This cuts
costs by dividing the same amount of work among a smaller pool
of people. Longer term, however, physicians who do nothing but
see patients every minute of the day will do little to secure medicine's future. Moreover, how feasible will it be to recruit and retain
physicians in academics when (1) we work as hard as community
practitioners and (2) we earn substantially less?

Certainly academic physicians need to account for academic
time. In this era of rapidly increasing clinical demands, no one
is suggesting that academic departments simply issue their
faculty members a blank check. Yet it would be equally fool-
hardy indiscriminately to reclaim as much non-clinical time as
possible. Recognizing the threat posed by its erosion, astute
leaders will seek out ways to enable academic physicians to
push the envelope of science and technology, to enhance understanding and respect for medicine among patients and other
health professionals, and to develop the leadership capacities
on which medicine's future depends. Doing so is one of the best
investments any academic department can make.

***

The future of medicine and the welfare of our patients hinge
on the quality of our leaders. Medicine's leaders are like ships'
captains. Poor leadership threatens to sink healthcare organizations. Mediocre leadership may leave us merely treading
water. Only good leadership will enable us to sail successfully
to our destinations. As we contemplate medicine's future, one
of the most promising investments we can make is to cultivate
the knowledge and skills of our future leaders, preparing them

to meet the challenges and opportunities that lie ahead. Yet many capable medical students, residents, and newly minted independent practitioners pay leadership little heed. Arrested leadership development may be traced in part to widely prevalent misconceptions or fallacies about leadership. We need to reflect on and discuss seven particularly debilitating leadership fallacies and what can be done about them.

The first leadership fallacy concerns the relevance of leadership. Some very intelligent, highly skilled, and dedicated people believe that leadership has little or nothing to do with us. We see ourselves as future clinicians, or scientists, or educators, but not as leaders. We have spent hundreds or even thousands of hours studying anatomy, pathology, medical technology, history taking, differential diagnosis, and therapeutics. We see ourselves as experts in these areas and continue to study such subjects throughout our careers, in an effort to remain on top of our field.

Yet we enjoyed little or no opportunity during medical school, residency, or continuing medical education to study leadership. We tend to see leadership as the province of business school graduates and politicians. To many of us, it is a black box. Leaders seem to us like the Wizard of Oz, mysteriously manipulating organizations' levers from behind a curtain. Viewing leadership as a black box creates serious problems. If many of the best junior people see leadership in these terms, who will be prepared to play leadership roles? In many cases, it is inevitable that future leaders will be drawn from the ranks of the less qualified.

More likely, leadership of hospitals and healthcare organizations will continue to shift to business school graduates. Many of these people have little or no experience in patient care, medical research, or medical education. In this scenario, the people deciding what equipment to purchase, whom to hire, and how to formulate budget and strategy will not understand the relationships between patients and health professionals from the inside. This may impact medicine and healthcare in ways that undermine effectiveness and fulfillment, and compromise the achievement of their core missions.

Leadership is not an esoteric topic relevant to a select few, but a ubiquitous feature of daily life for every physician. Every clinician is a leader of a team of colleagues comprised of other physicians, nurses, clerical staff, and so on. Every educator is a leader of medical students and residents. Every parent is a leader of children. Every person who bears any responsibility in an organization is a leader, at least in so far as we influence how the work gets done. Even those of us who think of ourselves as followers are leaders. People in positions of greater formal authority depend on us for an understanding of what is happening in the organization. In shaping the perceptions of leaders, we function as leaders on our own right.

In many organizations, people with the most formal authority do not necessarily exert the most influence. In meetings, for example, it is not always the person who presides who most shapes others' opinions. Even a very junior person can wield a great deal of influence by expressing important ideas well. In short, leaders are not so rare as we sometimes suppose. Far rarer, in fact, are individuals who enjoy no opportunity to lead.

Another disabling fallacy concerns the lack of leadership qualifications. Many otherwise capable people fear that we lack what it takes to be a leader. As a result, when opportunities to lead present themselves, we duck and cover, hoping that someone else will step forward to shoulder the responsibility. This is a venerable theme in Western culture. In the Bible, God recruits Moses to go to Pharaoh and tell him to release the people of Israel from bondage (Fig. 6.1). The reluctant Moses responds, "Who am I to go to Pharaoh, and that I should bring the children of Israel out of Egypt?" Later, as God tells him how this will be accomplished, Moses expresses doubts about his ability to convince the Israelites to follow him: "But suppose they will not believe me or listen to my voice?" A bit later, Moses again resists, saying "I am not eloquent, neither before nor since you have spoken to your servant; I am slow of speech and slow of tongue." Finally, Moses reluctantly agrees to serve as God's spokesperson, but only with the stipulation that his silver-tongued brother, Aaron, will address the people for him.

Many of us operate with the mistaken notion that leaders are born and not made. Having known few successful leadership experiences in our lives and recognizing that people do not

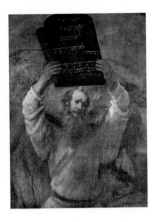

Fig. 6.1 Rembrandt's *Moses with the Tablets* (1659). Moses not only led the Israelites out of bondage in Egypt but also served as their most important lawgiver. Though he represented one of the most important leaders in the Judeo-Christian tradition, Moses initially assumed the mantle of leadership only with great reluctance

seem to turn to us in times of crisis, we suppose that we are missing a crucial set of genes that makes some people innately effective leaders. In meetings, we are not the first to speak up. We do not feel compelled to ensure that our will always prevails. We are not the life of every cocktail party, and groups of people do not necessarily coalesce around us in social settings. Perhaps we have been disappointed by the few formal leadership opportunities that came our way or found the experience baffling or unrewarding, or even a failure.

In fact, however, effective leaders need not be the tallest, or best looking, or most naturally congenial people. They are not necessarily the best conversationalists, nor would they necessarily be voted the most popular. Many effective leaders, such as Abraham Lincoln, have been rather private, shy, and even self-conscious people. Leadership is more of an art than an ability. People are born with abilities, including abilities in different arts. For example, some people have a knack for musicianship, others for art, others for mathematics, and still others for simple congeniality. Yet even more important than sheer ability are such factors such as how hard we work at cultivating our innate talents, how strongly we wish to excel at what we do, and above all, how much we care about the people we work with.

Even people with many natural gifts for leadership fail. We fail because we do not understand what the organization should be trying to do. Plato once wrote that power should be entrusted only to people who are not in love with it. Why? Because people who are in love with power may not care about what happens to other people in the organization or about achieving the organization's missions. Instead, we simply want to be in charge. There is something reassuring about Moses' attitude. He did not set out to lead. Instead, he doubted that he was qualified for the job. It was only as he came to understand the importance of the goal toward which leadership was needed that he became a great leader. For Moses, knowledge of the good came before the desire to lead. With time and experience, he grew into a role he was not initially prepared to play. Those of us who recognize opportunities to lead should spend less time worrying about our lack of qualifications and more time trying to understand where our organizations need to go.

Another leadership fallacy concerns the nature of leadership. Many people suppose that the most important measure of leaders is our ability to get other people to do what we want. The further we can move others from where they want to go, the more effective we are as leaders. Leadership, in other words, is conceptualized in terms of influence. What means could leaders employ to exert influence? One approach would be persuasion, using reasoned argument to try to convince people that it lies in everyone's interest to pursue a different goal. Yet other less noble approaches might work, too. For example, withholding information, or even outright deception, might help to change others' minds. Similarly, bribing people might change their priorities. So might coercion, threatening people with the loss of their jobs.

As these examples indicate, leadership is not about getting people to do what we want. Bullies and extortionists may be able to impose their will on others, but no one would call a bully or an extortionist a leader. Instead leadership is about helping people to see what we ought to want because it is best for us, or best for our organization, or best for the people the organization serves. Merely getting people to do what we want is the definition of tyranny. How do tyrants think about the needs and aspirations of others? In most cases, they see others as tools for the satisfaction of their own desires. They regard them as the buttons and levers they need to manipulate to get what they want. When people fail to follow orders, they are quite prepared to do away with them because they are not interested in people. They could hardly care less about colleagues, so long as they get what they want.

True leaders, by contrast, really care about the people we work with and want to see them happy and fulfilled in the work they do. Really caring about other people as people, and not merely as cogs in a machine, means refraining from shouting at them like tyrants, and instead talking with them. Above all, it means listening to them. We should recognize that a two-way flow of information is vital if we are to understand our organization and the people who make it up. True leaders are not so much dictators as learners, always seeking to understand our colleagues and putting this understanding to work in the life of the organization.

Is leadership a matter of technique? From a technician's point of view, what matters most about leadership is how we lead. Should we be open with people or secretive? Should we be readily available to meet with people on a moment's notice or difficult to reach? Should we deal with people through intermediaries or face to face? Should we delegate most of our authority or attempt to do as much as possible ourselves? These are the questions that preoccupy a leadership technician. There is no doubt that some approaches to leadership are more fruitful than others. Yet the role of technique tends to be over-emphasized. Whether we are traveling by air, sea, rail, or road, it is more important to understand where we are headed than how we are getting there. In order to know how to travel, we must first define our destination.

Knowing how to lead requires knowing where the organization should be headed. Merely moving quickly and efficiently is no advantage if we are moving in the wrong direction. In other words, leadership techniques need to be adapted to the challenges and opportunities at hand. The approach that works best when things are going well may not be well suited to a crisis. So, too, different leadership approaches are called for, depending on the colleagues with whom responsibility can be shared. Good leaders focus on the goals first and the technique second. Courses on leadership tend to focus too much on technique, in part because techniques are relatively easy to teach. For example, it is easy to teach participants different techniques for brainstorming, or ranking priorities, or delivering bad news. Harder but much more important is educating people to better define what our priorities ought to be. To do this, it is not sufficient merely to master a technique. Our need for leadership techniques is far exceeded by our need to understand ourselves, our colleagues, our organizations, and the changing environments in which we are situated.

It would be unfortunate if people could seize power in an organization simply by mastering techniques we learned at a weekend seminar. Like most important things in life, earning the prerogative of leadership and excelling as a leader require serious effort. There are no short cuts to understanding what an organization should strive to become.

One of the most seductive features of leadership is the prestige associated with it. There is a natural tendency to suppose that people in positions of leadership are the best. We look at the higher compensation, larger offices, special privileges, greater authority, and enhanced access to information that leaders enjoy and suppose that being placed in a leadership position instantly makes a person a big shot. Nothing could be further from the truth. The people who get the corner office often do not last long. In some cases, the fault lies not with the newly appointed leader, but with the dire situation into which the leader was placed. Moreover, the prestige associated with leadership can undermine relationships with colleagues, rendering them shallow and even artificial. Prestige can also become a distraction, so entrancing us that we lose track of the reasons we wanted to lead in the first place.

Good leaders do not spend much time looking in the mirror. There is no room for selfishness. Good leaders regard knowledge, skill, and experience as tools with which to serve. Our first commitment should be not to ourselves, but to the mission of the organization we lead. If we seek authority, it should not be to make ourselves look bigger, but to make a contribution. Our goal is to make a difference in the life of the organization and the people who work in it. We want to know that the organization would suffer if we were not there. We want to play an important role in forming teams, helping teams thrive, and enabling colleagues to perform at their best. The desire for authority is not a bad thing. So long as we intend to use it for the appropriate purposes, it is a good thing. It would spell trouble for organizations if no one cared enough about us to want to serve.

Really good leaders can make leadership look easy. Faced with a difficult situation, they best seem to know instinctively what to do to diffuse tension, or cut through the fog, or jump-start a stalling project. In fact, however, effective leadership is not easy. It is like practicing medicine. A medical student watching a physician examine a patient might conclude that medicine takes little effort, because the physician can form an accurate diagnostic impression in only a few minutes. In fact, however, good physicians have invested years or even decades of effort to be able to make such rapid and apparently effortless assessments.

To become a good leader requires a great deal of effort to get to know the organization, the people in it, and the environment in which it operates. What seems like a spur-of-the-moment, instinctive stroke of brilliance in fact requires long study of the organization's priorities and its style of operation. Only people who really care about our organizations and work hard to learn as much as we can about them will be in a position to succeed.

A famous example of a leader who made it look easy was Sir Winston Churchill (Fig. 6.2), one of the most important political leaders of the twentieth century and a Nobel Laureate

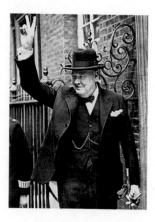

Fig. 6.2 Sir Winston Churchill (1874–1965), one of the greatest statesmen and orators of the twentieth century, who led the British people during one of their darkest hours. In 1953, he also won the Nobel Prize in Literature for "his mastery of historical and biographical descriptions as well as for brilliant oratory in defending exalted human values"

in Literature. Churchill was also known as one of the century's great orators, having achieved worldwide fame for such memorable utterances as: "Never in the field of human conflict was so much owed by so many to so few," "We shall draw from the heart of suffering itself the means of inspiration and survival," and "Let us therefore brace ourselves to our duty, and so bear ourselves that, if the British Empire and its Commonwealth lasts for a thousand years, men will still say, 'This was their finest hour.'" Listening to Churchill's famous radio broadcasts during the Second World War or witnessing his speeches in person, many people had the impression that he spoke extemporaneously and was simply an extraordinarily gifted speaker. However, we know from Churchill's own writings that he worked for hours, sometimes days, to formulate what he would say, and practiced his speeches many times over. In fact, Churchill was a stutterer, and he struggled with a speech impediment his entire life.

Perhaps the greatest leadership fallacy is the notion that accepting formal leadership responsibility means sacrificing the other things in life we really care about. Must great leaders give up all pretense of maintaining a happy family life? Must leaders set aside personal ambitions for clinical work, research, and education to such a degree that we lose ourselves in our organizations? Must those of us who aspire to formal leadership positions be prepared to relinquish even our own moral scruples for the good of the organization? These are very dangerous misconceptions, partly because they inevitably turn good people away from leadership. If playing a formal leadership role means wrecking our personal life, abandoning the professional challenges that attracted us to medicine in the first place, and even being forced to do things that trouble our conscience, then who wants it?

Far from diminishing a person, however, leadership provides wonderful opportunities for personal development through service. Excelling as a leader requires the development of many of the most important human virtues, such as courage, self-control, compassion, justice, moral discernment, and wisdom. To become a great leader requires sustained personal growth and satisfies the human need to serve a purpose larger than ourselves. Instead of abandoning what we care most about, leadership invites us to pursue it to an even greater extent. We should try to make our organizations places where people can flourish both personally and professionally. Ideally, everyone, including leaders, should feel fully engaged in what the organization does. There is no reason that even chairs should not continue to devote some time and energy to former professional pursuits. Continued clinical work and/or scholarly activity helps leaders remain more in touch with the life of the faculty and better acquainted with the day-to-day activities of the organization.

Above all, prospective leaders should not assume that we must check our moral and religious convictions at the portal of leadership. It is simply not the case that only Machiavellian types need apply. One of the hallmarks of great leaders is a moral vision for the organization, one that places integrity and commitment to high principles at the core of organizational life. No matter how clever, urbane, and politically adroit we might be, great leadership is not possible absent such moral vision.

It is vital that physicians at every stage of professional development pause from time to time to reflect on leadership. Talented people who never saw ourselves as leadership material need to discover the hidden leader within. People who already aspire to formal leadership need to deepen our understanding of what it means to be a leader, and what leaders need to do to promote the flourishing of our organizations. People who occupy leadership positions need to reexamine our leadership performance and seek out opportunities to perform even better. Departments and national professional organizations need to recognize the importance of fostering future leaders and to develop and refine leadership programs. Even people who think of ourselves primarily as followers need to reexamine what we expect from leaders and consider what we might contribute to make leaders more effective. Above all, we need to recognize, study, and effectively respond to the fallacies that lead leaders and potential leaders astray.

Chapter 7
Effective Leadership

When it comes to leading academic medicine, we should take more of our cues from the biological sciences. After all, clinical medicine represents applied human biology, and medicine is deeply rooted in biological theories and techniques. A biological approach contrasts sharply with a mechanistic model, which treats the academic health center as an assembly line. Assembly lines tend to be efficient but impersonal, with little interaction between the people who work on them. What is the level of interaction in contemporary medical education between the basic medical sciences and clinical medicine, primary care and specialty care, students and faculty, faculty and administration, and the medical school and the community in which it is situated? At the very least, it could be improved. A biological approach can open up between these areas new opportunities for synergy, enhancing the quality of work we do. The seeds of synergy are present, but to reap their fruits we need to sow them more effectively.

We can treat boundaries less as barriers and more as breeding grounds. Students, faculty members, and administrators can function less as border guards and more as ambassadors. Academic health centers need not be organized into departmental and disciplinary silos. We can start viewing them as interdependent habitats. We can transform medical schools into genuine communities of discovery, which serve as catalysts for transformation throughout our institutions of higher learning. To do so, we need to explore an important biological concept: the ecotone.

R.B. Gunderman, *Leadership in Healthcare*,
DOI 10.1007/978-1-84800-943-1_7,
© Springer-Verlag London Limited 2009

An ecotone is an area where two or more adjacent habitats meet and commingle. Examples include the interface between a grassland and a desert or between a lake and a forest. Such areas tend to manifest great richness and diversity, often displaying substantially more biological dynamism than the habitats they border. In them are species native to the adjoining habitats, as well as species distinct to the ecotones themselves, whose marginal status fosters the development of new biological capabilities. Because ecotones exhibit the greatest biological ferment, they are among the most fruitful sites for ecological study.

There are two fundamentally different ways to think about ecotones: as threats or opportunities. Viewed as threats, ecotones seem to be the sites of the most vicious biological competition. In them, species strain against one another in the face of conditions far more perilous than they might encounter nestled in the core of their habitat. If security alone were the living world's greatest reward, then most organisms might do better to steer clear of ecotones.

Yet ecotones are also prodigious engines of biological innovation. Diversity and dynamism are at their greatest on the margins, between habitats. Here whole new biological forms originate. For example, new structures such as legs and lungs probably first developed in marine organisms living in shallow pools near land. Had such creatures remained in deep water, such structures would have conferred no biological advantage. Ecotones are not necessarily places where organisms must kill or be killed. Many ecotonal interactions are more cooperative and even synergistic than antagonistic.

The word ecotone is derived from Greek. The stem *eco-*, which contributes to our words economics and ecology, means "house." To ancient Greeks such as Aristotle, economics referred to the art and science of managing a household. Today ecology refers to the study of the relationships between different living organisms and their biological domains. The root *tonos* is the source of our word tone and means "string" or "to stretch." Tones were the sounds generated by plucking the strings of a musical instrument. If violins and pianos are to produce their characteristic tones, their strings cannot be lax. To make music, they must be stretched taut. An ecotone, then, is a place where biological habitats, the home turfs of different organisms and species, are stretched to their limit.

In biology as in economics, risk and reward are closely correlated. Ecotones challenge the creatures who inhabit them, but they also open up opportunities for the development of new capabilities and the forging of new relationships. Many innovations fail, but those that succeed often do so spectacularly. The biological capacities for vision and flight represented huge gambles, but for some organisms they have paid off extraordinarily handsomely.

The history of science furnishes numerous examples of ecotones' vital role in innovation. Many of the most important biological discoveries of the twentieth century were the work not of biologists, but scientists addressing biological problems from the vantage points of other disciplines. The structure and function of DNA were unlocked largely by applying theories and techniques from physics and chemistry. Again and again, major scientific advances spring from people who look at a discipline's problems from the outside. As Einstein famously declared, "We cannot solve problems by using the same kind of thinking we used when we created them."

This is not to say that we should do away with cultural, intellectual, and scientific boundaries. We cannot simply blend disciplines together in a large pot. For human life to develop, distinct biomolecules had to aggregate to produce organelles, organelles had to aggregate to produce cells, distinct cell types had to aggregate to produce tissues, and distinct tissues had to aggregate to produce specialized organs. Life depends on the presence of interfaces across which chemical, electrical, and molecular gradients can be sustained. To break down such interfaces would forfeit not only specialization but life itself. Biologists have a word for a state of complete equilibrium: death.

Yet life in isolation carries a great price for cells, organisms, species, and ecosystems. Nearly every living cell in the human body is located within a hundred microns of a capillary. If cells were not in such close proximity to the bloodstream, nutrients and waste products could not be exchanged at a sufficient rate to sustain life. Isolation is also a recipe for reproductive failure. To realize the full benefits of sexual reproduction, mating must take place between genetically dissimilar organisms. Isolation produces inbreeding, which undermines biological fitness by aggregating harmful genes. By comparison, hybrids exhibit enhanced biological vigor and resiliency.

There are many ecotones in academic medicine. These include interfaces between primary care and tertiary care, faculty and students, and the scientific and ethical aspects of medicine.

Ecologists ask certain questions about ecotones. One concerns their origin. From an institutional point of view, the science/ethics interface might seem to have sprung up with the arrival of professional ethicists just a few decades ago, when courses in medical ethics first began to appear in medical school curricula. In fact, however, the interface between science and ethics is an intrinsic feature of medicine, as old as the profession itself. Without science, we could not develop ventilators, but without ethical judgment, we could not tell when to use them and when to turn them off.

Aristotle held that medicine consists of both theoretical and practical dimensions. Theoretically, the same scientific knowledge that enables physicians to promote health could also be used to harm patients. Pharmacology provides physician/scientists with the know-how to end life as well as preserve it. Practically speaking, however, medicine includes a commitment to the promotion of patient welfare. A physician necessarily labors on behalf of health. The interface between science and ethics may shift from time to time, but it will never disappear from medicine. External forces also shape and sustain the science/ethics ecotone. Funding is one such force. The fact that the amount of research funding for molecular biology vastly exceeds that for healthcare ethics inevitably shapes the curricula of medical schools and the career choices of physicians.

Students at two different medical schools might develop widely divergent views of the relationship between biomedical science and ethics based on very different educational experiences. Suppose the first school sees its mission as educating primary care clinicians. It emphasizes medicine's artful side, while teaching only the fundamentals of the basic medical sciences. By contrast, the second school aims above all to prepare basic science researchers. Its faculty members resist any effort to augment ethics in the curriculum, arguing that there is insufficient classroom time to cover just the science.

When we study the origins of ecotones, we realize that we have the capacity to shape many of them. There is little we can do about the Grand Canyon, but a great deal we could do about the Berlin Wall. Which of the interfaces of academic medicine are relatively fixed, and which can we revise? When it comes to how these latter interfaces are configured, is uniformity or diversity more desirable? From an ecological perspective, it makes more sense to allow different departments and schools to experiment and innovate, rather than force every one to conform to a single model. So long as academic medical centers share experiences, fostering diversity is the most fruitful approach.

Another important feature of ecotones is their structure. Structure can be examined through a number of different lenses. One is granularity. This refers to the vantage point from which we inspect an object, with our noses up against it or from a great distance. An object's appearance changes dramatically depending on the level of magnification. It is only when we view human tissues through a microscope that we discover that they are made up of cells. Yet if we view a newspaper photograph at progressively greater levels of magnification, soon we are able to perceive little more than a jumble of dots.

At what level of granularity should we examine the ecotones of academic medicine? Should we focus on the healthcare needs of our society, our vision of a well-educated physician, the distinctive mission of each particular medical school, or the teaching interests of faculty members who happen to populate each department? There is no requirement that we confine ourselves to a single level of granularity. A comprehensive view requires that we shift back and forth between multiple perspectives, just as a physician treating a patient shifts between psychosocial, cellular, and molecular perspectives. Academic medicine is like a Japanese pond: we must walk around to see all of it. No single perspective reveals everything.

Another key structural feature of ecotones is thickness. If the boundaries between medical disciplines are too wide, little or no interaction can take place between them. In this situation, students are likely to develop a compartmentalized, fragmented view of medicine that undermines the ability to integrate diverse perspectives in teaching, research, service, and clinical practice. If we paint the medical school and its community as isolated from one another by high walls and a deep moat, we should not be surprised when students evince little interest in community service or the social context of medicine.

Yet distinctions are important. Ecotones cannot be so thin that they provide no space for anything to happen. If the curriculum so tightly intertwines science and ethics that students never appreciate the distinctiveness of their approaches, their potential for synergism will be undermined. Who would savor the courses of a gourmet meal if they were all pureed together? The goal is not to dissolve all diversity of perspective, but to provide opportunities for distinct disciplines to interact productively. As the pace of discovery quickens, it becomes increasingly counterproductive to keep disciplines sealed off from one another. Students, faculty members, departments, institutions, and communities are rewarded less for insularity than for hybridization, and the structure of our organizations needs to reflect this. We need places to meet and talk to exchange ideas and perspectives.

Ecotones have not only spatial dimensions but also temporal dimensions. To achieve collaboration, we need meeting time as well as meeting space. If students feel they have no choice but to devote every available minute to memorizing the content of each course, many will never explore disciplinary interfaces. Physicians educated in such an environment are less likely to appreciate how scientific and ethical perspectives can join to promote patient welfare, or how academic physicians and civic leaders can work together to improve community health.

The principle of collaboration has both interpersonal and intrapersonal dimensions. Interpersonally, we need to permit students in different courses and phases of training to interact with one another. Student mentorship programs can be effective, as can regular social events. In the intrapersonal sphere, we need to provide time for students to step back and consider how different courses fit together.

Disciplines need to contact one another, and perhaps even overlap. Interfaces should be relatively translucent. It is rare that one department's work needs to be hidden from the others. A boat is unlikely to get very far if none of the rowers knows what the others are doing. Such sequestration promotes myopia, undermining collaboration. Each department should feel free to explore the work of others, helping to develop a clearer sense of where the institution as a whole is headed. Faculty members representing different disciplines could give lectures or lead discussions in one another's courses, or even team teach.

A related issue is the integrity of interfaces. No cell could survive if its membranes became impermeable. Academic medical centers need to think of the interfaces between departments like the semi-permeable membranes of living cells. We can thrive only if our disciplinary boundaries are perforated, permitting the fruitful exchange of ideas and perspectives. Too much permeability and we lapse into lifeless equilibrium. Too little permeability and we die from lack of nutrients or drown in the toxic byproducts of our own metabolism. We cannot afford to see academic medical centers as fiefdoms and fortresses, focused primarily on security and the preservation of the status quo. We need departments that are open, outward looking, and attuned to innovation and collaboration.

Ecotones have shapes. In some cases, such as the glass walls of an aquarium, the interface is perfectly straight, and the transition very abrupt. In other cases, the border is more complex. Consider the surface of the human small intestine, whose plicae circularis, villi, and microvilli multiply the bowel's absorptive surface area several hundred fold. In academic medicine as in biology, straight lines and abrupt transitions are ineffective at promoting interchange and collaboration. Interdigitated borders are far more fruitful.

Relationships between disciplines may be situated at any one of a number of different points along a continuum. Faculty members and students in each discipline may be mutually antagonistic, each seeing the other as a drain on valuable resources. They may be ignorant of one another. They may tolerate one another. Or they may actively cooperate. The most fruitful relationship between disciplines is one of synergism, in which each actively enhances the work of the other and that of the organization as a whole.

Biology provides innumerable examples of synergism. One is the relationship between the once independent prokaryotic organisms that became mitochondria and the now eukaryotic cells in which they took up permanent residence. The larger cells gained metabolic powerhouses, while the smaller cells received shelter and nutrients. This instance of endosymbiosis is thought to have occurred approximately two billion years ago. Another more recent example of synergism is the commensal relationship between human beings and the bacteria that normally inhabit our gut. The microorganisms gain shelter and nutrients, while the host benefits from a reliable supply of vitamin K and assistance keeping more pernicious microorganisms at bay.

How could we promote greater synergism among the ecotones of academic medicine? To begin with, we need to consider the range of roles they might play. In nature, some ecotones function in a largely absorptive fashion. For example, when whales are washed up on shore by a rapidly receding tide, they are absorbed by the land. Contributions from one habitat are simply swallowed up by another, and no innovation occurs. Reflection is another outcome of separating habitats by an impermeable membrane. It occurs at the glass walls of an aquarium, or the edge of a lake. Fish can brush up against and even collide with the interface, but they cannot penetrate it. Examples in academic medicine include faculty members who never attend conferences outside their own discipline. If absorption or reflection most typifies our boundary interactions, academic medicine is in peril.

A somewhat more productive role is transmission. An example of transmission is the flooding of a river, which conveys fish to new ponds and lakes. In academic medicine, a transmitter can contribute in modest ways by regulating the speed and quantity of ideas that pass from one domain to another, helping to prevent both shortage and excess. A still more fruitful role is intensification. This occurs when the messenger not only transmits the message but also actually enhances it in some way. For example, if a clinician describes to medical students how knowing a scientific principle enhances the care of a patient, the principle may become more meaningful and memorable to the students. Conversely, a basic scientist may show students how a particular clinical case beautifully exemplifies a scientific principle.

The most fruitful role of ecotones is usually transformation. In this case, messengers serve as active creators in their own right. Disciplines engage in active dialogue with one another, generating new questions, insights, and collaborative endeavors. Such dialogue can occur both intramurally, within the walls of medical schools, and extramurally, through partnerships with other schools, public health groups, corporations, government, and so on. The situation is like that of an orchestra at rest. All of the musical instruments are there, each well maintained and tuned. The challenge to the conductor is to get the musicians playing together in symphonic harmony.

Medical schools can be strong intellectual presences in our universities. Why should not academic medicine blaze a trail of interdisciplinary collaboration? Why should not the medical school be the most exciting conversation on campus? Faculty and administrative offices can function not as fortresses but as embassies, with different disciplines strategically positioned in close proximity to one another. Some classrooms can be configured not as lecture halls but as seminar rooms, permitting learning to take place conversationally. Because informal meeting space is no less important than formal space, lounges, dining halls, and even recreation facilities can foster interdisciplinary exchange,.

Interdisciplinary teaching and research are vital. We need to offer truly grand rounds in which faculty members and students from different disciplines participate on a regular basis. Interdisciplinary collaborations should be tracked and publicized. Faculty, students, and administrators should be recruited and rewarded in part for interdisciplinary activity. Examples might include a research collaboration between a molecular biologist and a infectious disease specialist, a teaching collaboration between a psychiatrist and a pediatrician, and a community service collaboration between a group of medical students and the members of a civic organization.

Critical to the concept of the ecotone is a favorable disposition toward knowledge sharing. Too many incentives in academic medicine point in the opposite direction, toward knowledge hoarding. We fear that if we share what we know, its value will diminish. In fact, however, most of what we know realizes its full value only when we put it to work in collaboration with others. New ideas are far more likely to emerge from knowledge sharing than knowledge hoarding. This does not mean that we should send all our data to colleagues in other disciplines. It does mean asking one another hard questions and testing our most basic assumptions. Some of the steps we need to take to enhance academic medicine have not even occurred to us.

The goal is to build bridges between our fields, challenge one another, and set new ideas in motion. Existing interfaces need to be both more porous and more fluid. It is less important that students take self-contained courses in disciplines such as physiology, pathology, internal medicine, and surgery than that they develop the capacity to excel as clinicians, educators, researchers, and leaders. The final product should not be determined by a curricular tug-of-war between the disciplines. Instead, the curriculum should be shaped by a comprehensive and rich vision of medical excellence. To achieve such a vision, we need to work together, developing the academic medical center as a laboratory of ideas. The best ideas will be generated not asexually but sexually. The future vitality of academic medicine rests on our ability to foster intercourse, recombination, and hybrid vigor.

Which inhabitants of the academic medical center exhibit the greatest unrealized fecundity? While faculty members and administrators have great potential, the greatest hope of all may lie with the students. They are not data repositories, vast memory banks. They are gifted human beings with untapped reservoirs of creativity and insight. Students encounter the medical schools' full range of disciplines, and see firsthand how different pathways intersect. Who is better situated to recombine disciplines in new and creative ways? Given the opportunity, they can do more than merely move from classroom to classroom. They can enhance our fertility, like bees pollinating fields of flowers. By cross fertilizing our disciplines, they can spark innovation and play a vital role in helping to promote synergism.

Some faculty members and administrators cross some disciplinary interfaces, but only the students move back and forth across all of them. What sorts of interdisciplinary projects can students devise, and how can we organize medical schools to foster such creative activities? We might think of students as human catalysts, lowering the energy of activation necessary for reagents to react with one another to produce a new compound. Yet the analogy with catalysts holds only to a point, for unlike catalysts, the students transform themselves in the process.

We should aim less to instruct students than to liberate students, to free them and enable them to stretch to their full potential. This is the true meaning of liberal education, one that prepares students to make their own informed judgments and to choose freely for themselves. They are no longer slaves to the past, simply parroting what they have been told. Now they can truly think and speak on their own. Moreover, their deepened understanding and compassion prepare them to give for the benefit of others.

To promote liberal education in medicine, the boundaries between us cannot be invisible fences that we dare not transgress. They must be frontiers that beckon us to exploration. Students should appreciate the benefits of looking at medicine from multiple perspectives and develop a broad intellectual foundation on which to build their lives. The way to a rich and fulfilling career is not isolation. Instead we need to interweave ourselves as deeply as possible into the tapestries of medicine and human life.

We need an increasing number of specialists to meet the healthcare needs of our communities, but medicine need not lapse into disconnected specialization. We need to develop increasingly sophisticated technology of diagnosis and treatment, but we need not become mere technicians. Medicine is above all a human science and a human art, and we need to ensure that the people we educate to practice it are able to draw on the full range of human learning. They need not be the most knowledge-able people in any particular discipline, but they should be among the most liberally educated and well rounded of all professionals, with the strongest commitment to the service of humanity.

The wider and deeper the ecotones in academic medicine, the greater the diversity of the faculty who will be attracted to them, and the richer the quality of interdisciplinary discourse and collaboration that will emerge from them. Life at the margins truly is the most fruitful. To promote this fertility, we need to foster more porous disciplinary and curricular interfaces, greater interdigitation of teaching and research activities, more dynamism across disciplines, and greater interaction between academic medical centers, universities, and communities. We especially need to look for opportunities to liberate academic medicine's most important ecotonal species, the medical students. With their help, we can ensure that academic medical centers and universities amount to more than the mere sum of their parts.

***

The governance of professional organizations is vital. Significant challenges confront the medical profession, warranting urgent attention. If professional organizations are to react with sufficient speed, vigor, and acumen to meet these challenges, we must ensure that the selection of leaders is a democratic and participatory process. It is now more important than ever that we avoid allowing leadership to become a largely honorific or ceremonial posting requiring little grasp of the challenges and opportunities facing the profession. Leadership must never be regarded as a mere sinecure that naturally devolves to individuals after long and distinguished careers. In a time when adaptability and innovation are called for, professional organizations must avoid the tendency to play it safe by controlling the process from above. We must avoid selecting candidates who have never attempted to offer a vision of the profession's future.

One of the most important functions of elections is to enable members to choose. When only one slate of candidates is offered, there is no choice. A lack of a meaningful choice can leave members feeling disengaged from the organization. Such a system of governance is more characteristic of the former Soviet Union than the United States. Professional organizations should strive to ensure that our elections provide members an opportunity to exercise genuine influence in the organization. The election of a leader should not become a mere formality, but provide a genuine choice between two more alternative views of the organization's mission, vision, strategic plan, and goals.

There is no question that a contested election can be awkward, generating lingering hard feelings among candidates and their groups of supporters. Yet few events more engage members in the life of an organization than an election where candidates sketch out who they are and what they stand for. Hearing candidates discuss the organization's future draws members into the debate, and gets us thinking about our own roles in achieving its objectives.

It is vital that the election process avoid assuming a "Wizard of Oz" character. In Oz, the person really controlling events stands behind a curtain, hidden from view, pulling levels, and turning dials. Were members to develop the sense that the selection of the organization's leaders is really the work of a group of wizards operating behind closed doors, our interest in playing an active role in the life of the organization would diminish. Like the citizens of the former Soviet Union, we would participate in the electoral process, if at all, only because we felt we had a duty to do so and not because we were engaged in directing the organization.

In such a scenario, members develop a sense of disengagement from the leadership, and leaders develop a sense of disengagement from the membership. Were aspiring leaders to realize that the members of the organization have very little influence over the process of leader selection, we would be less inclined to try to listen to what members have to say. If members were to develop the sense that the only contribution we make to the organization is to pay dues, many might begin to question the value of remaining a member.

A relatively closed, top-down model of organizational governance is a prescription for a passive, uninvolved membership and a conformist, paternalistic leadership. In the worst-case scenario, members would lose all interest in an organization over which we felt they had no influence. Leaders, in turn, would contribute to this downward spiral in democratic participation by beginning to think and act as though the organization existed for us, instead of we for the organization. We might even begin to make decisions based on what we thought was good for the leadership, as opposed to what was good for the organization as a whole. It is vital that professional organizations attempt actively to involve new members in governance. We must not spend our first years or even decades of membership in a purely passive frame of mind, playing the role of people for whom decisions are made, rather than people who play an active role in making decisions. By encouraging engagement in the electoral process, organizations can serve as breeding grounds for leadership, helping to develop the section chiefs, department chairs, hospital CEOs, and deans of tomorrow.

Elections should get members excited about what the organization is doing. They should be regarded as opportunities for leaders to enlist the members' vigorous support and cooperation in building the profession's future. Organizations should get candidates actively invested in the process, encouraging them to interact with members, and clearly to formulate and express their vision for the organization's future. Inevitably, mistakes will occur, but it is better to have candidates who attempt to craft a vision for the organization and fail than to have candidates who regard leadership as a sinecure to which they are entitled because they are next in line. It is also better than allowing the leadership of organizations to become highly inbred, with each new leader selected by past leaders, which can quickly render vision and strategy stale. In politics as in biology, mutation and recombination are salutary, because they foster creativity and tend to produce a more robust organization better adapted for success in a changing environment.

Elections should remain interesting and thought-provoking events that invite the input of the whole organization. They should never come to resemble jealously guarded invitations to join an elite "old boy network" extended by an elite group of "old boys." A far better metaphor would be a laboratory of ideas, where bright people are encouraged to put forward new visions and strategies for the organization's future. Organizations that adopt such an approach serve as leadership engines, fostering the development of leaders committed less to protecting the organization from change than to putting the organization at the forefront of innovation. This enables important challenges and opportunities to be recognized sooner, with more genuine discussion and debate over alternative responses, and positions the organization years ahead of the curve it would otherwise trace out. Junior members of such an organization view its leader selection process not as a black box, but as a transparent, stimulating process that beckons them to become involved. The leadership of the organization is not separated from the people whom it most needs to recruit and involve.

In sum, the challenges confronting medicine at the moment are simply too momentous to allow our national organizations to slip into bad habits of leader selection. A democratic system, even one that involves hotly contested elections, is better for the overall health of the profession than one in which this vital task is ceded to a leadership elite. The latter alternative may foster organizational stability, but it does so at the price of discouraging innovation. Moreover, it tends to limit both members' active participation in the life of the organization and the degree to which leaders feel responsible to the membership. A truly democratic process of leader selection produces better leaders and enhances the organization as a whole, by encouraging both members and leaders to discuss a vision for the profession and the organization's role in pursuing it. Elections are the single most important recurring opportunity to foster this type of discussion, and one we can ill afford to squander.

***

Knowledge sharing should represent a core competency of our academic institutions and a major commitment of our leaders. Yet as medicine has become increasingly specialized and academic medical centers have grown larger and more complex, the tendency for knowledge to be compartmentalized has grown apace. The greater the number and functional diversity of people in an organization, the more difficult it becomes to share knowledge. This problem afflicts not only academic medical centers but also the larger universities of which they are a part. What was once a university has, in many cases, become a multiversity, and the same could be said, to a lesser degree, for medical schools. Units function as silos, with relatively little meaningful interaction. This failure to share knowledge portends ill for academic medicine. Consider the following scenarios:

> Facing growing competition and declining reimbursements, an academic medical center makes several sweeping business decisions, including an alliance with a large for-profit hospital chain. Within three years, the academic medical center is insolvent, and teaching programs for medical students and residents suffer serious cutbacks. In reviewing events, a new dean discovers that numerous faculty members foresaw these difficulties, but their voices were not heard. They had never been consulted by the previous administration, which preferred to minimize the number of people involved in high-level decision-making.

> An academic department graduates residents who are well prepared for clinical practice, but almost none of its graduates choose academic careers. In an effort to determine why, the residency director interviews a number of the residents. They report that they receive no virtually instruction or mentorship in research and teaching, and no one has ever spoken with them about the advantages of an academic career.

> In an effort to increase an academic department's extramural research funding, a new dean introduces a performance-based

compensation system for faculty. This new system apportions a fixed pool of salary bonuses among researchers according to their extramural grant support. Over several years, the chairman observes a sharp decline in the quality of interdisciplinary collaboration between departments, as well as a lower overall level of extramural funding. When asked why, researchers report that the new system penalizes them for sharing what they know with "competitors" from other departments.

A department loses two of its most valued nurses over a period of several months. Upon looking into the matter, the chairman discovers that a new faculty member is partly to blame. The nurses regard this individual as difficult to work with. After counseling the new faculty member, staff relations improve, but it takes over a year to fill the nursing vacancies, during which time clinical operations suffer. Why did not the nurses voice their concerns? They suspected that their complaints would be ignored and feared that expressing them would simply cast them as malcontents.

When physicians and medical organizations fail to share knowledge effectively, both groups perform below their potential. This failure can undermine everything a department does, from teaching to research, patient care, and service. Only by reexamining academic medical organizations in light of the value of knowledge sharing can we achieve the level of excellence possible in true communities of learning and practice. This article traces out some of the impediments to knowledge sharing within and among academic medical centers, highlights the advantages of moving to organizational models that resemble communities more than silos, and outlines some basic strategies leaders can pursue to bring this about.

In some respects, academic physicians and medical schools are good at sharing knowledge. Teaching, which necessarily involves knowledge sharing, represents a primary commitment of many academic physicians. Likewise, research productivity is measured in terms of public presentations and publications. In academic medicine, both teaching and research promote the dissemination of information. Yet true knowledge sharing does not consist of a mere transfer of information. It involves the give and take of ideas, reasoned argument, and active collaboration in the pursuit of better understanding. True knowledge sharing is what universities should be all about.

Certain features of academic medicine actually discourage knowledge sharing. Beginning in the earliest years of premedical education, achievement tends to be defined at the individual level. Students take tests, earn grades, and gain admission to medical school as individuals. Once they matriculate in medical school, they continue to compete with one another for academic recognition and residency positions. After training, academic physicians are hired, promoted, and rewarded largely on an individual basis. To this focus on individual achievement, medicine adds a strong evaluative bias toward cognitive performance. People are rewarded primarily for the expression of what they know, and we tend to think that the best medical students, house officers, and faculty members are the ones who know the most. In light of the pervasiveness of these perspectives, it should come as no surprise that physicians develop attitudes that undermine the sharing of knowledge. "If I tell my colleagues everything I know," they may think, "how can I possibly look good by comparison?"

In the industrial age, the competitive view of knowledge and the top-down style of management it spawned made a certain amount of sense. Each individual on an assembly line had a defined task that changed very little from day to day or year to year, and instructions for carrying out a job could be specified prospectively and in detail. Little initiative and creativity were required to do the job well, and individual workers were rewarded simply for accomplishing their assigned tasks. They merely needed to put the same nut on the same bolt in the same way every time, a task at which many were eventually supplanted by robots. The job of figuring out what to build and how to build it could be left to a group of higher-level managers, who wielded the real knowledge on which the organization depended.

In this system, tangible assets constituted the means of production. Land, raw materials, and equipment appeared to be the crucial ingredients for success. One important feature of tangible assets is a tendency to diminish when shared. A farmer who shares part of his land with someone else produces lower yields himself, and a worker who allows others to use his equipment sees his personal productivity fall. By contrast, the information age places a premium not on tangible assets but on intangible assets. In terms of productivity, people are defined less by what we have than by what we know. In this setting, the distribution of knowledge is not a zero-sum game, in which one person's gain is another person's loss. Workers can share knowledge, unlike land or a piece of machinery, without diminishing it.

Academic medicine has always been a highly knowledge-intensive field, where efforts to impose an industrial model of production are doomed to fail. Many of the strategies by which industrial organizations once attempted to increase output simply do not work where intangible means of production such as knowledge are concerned. There is a fundamental difference between increasing the rate at which an assembly line produces automobiles and increasing the rate at which a group of academic physicians generates good ideas. On the assembly line, workers are functioning in series, the output of each limited by the others' rate of production. In a knowledge-generating environment, workers are functioning not in series but in parallel. The velocity, quantity, and quality of output all hinge on the interactions between the group's members, the degree of cooperation they achieve.

In contrast to the assembly line, caring for patients, creating new biomedical knowledge, and educating the next generation of physicians require significant investments of initiative and creativity by frontline workers. Each patient is different, each discovery requires a different approach, and the content of teaching is constantly changing. Tools such as clinical algorithms and practice guidelines can add value, but to develop and apply such tools appropriately requires insights that cannot be formalized in procedure manuals and imposed uniformly across an organization. Especially in today's rapidly changing healthcare environment, organizations optimize their chances of success not by telling physicians what to do, but by enabling them to make well-informed choices.

No single health professional knows everything he or she needs to know. As a result, failure to share knowledge compromises performance. Ineffective routines are continued, new approaches go unexplored, and opportunities to improve efficiency get overlooked, simply because we make decisions from needlessly constrained perspectives. Often the problem is not that the requisite knowledge cannot be found within the organization, but that faculty members fail to share what we know. As a result, some people do not appreciate what we need to know, while others do not recognize the value of the knowledge we possess. Often the explicit knowledge captured in an organization's rules and databases is less important than the implicit knowledge reflected in our goals, and our grasp of what is and is not possible.

Where the sharing of knowledge is concerned, the key performance parameter is not velocity or efficiency in any narrowly quantifiable sense. Instead, the key is synergy, literally "working together." When we truly work together, the whole is greater than the sum of its parts, because each individual in a group offers a distinctive perspective that no other member can duplicate. Each knows things, draws on experiences, and perceives problems and opportunities that others do not. When everyone shares these perspectives, the group as a whole is able to develop better informed, more creative approaches to the problems we face. To be sure, when groups are dominated by narrow-minded individuals, or adopt ineffective patterns of interaction, we tend to perform poorly. Yet when the members of a group are able to cooperate effectively, the group as a whole typically outperforms every individual member.

Though often touted as a way to enhance knowledge sharing, reliance on technology can prove counterproductive. Data can be stored and manipulated out in cyberspace, but knowledge can only be shared between living, breathing human beings. A computer can do the number-crunching work of hundreds of people, yet even the most sophisticated and expensive information technology ever devised cannot substitute for the insight, judgment, and creativity of bright and committed human beings. At its deepest level, real knowledge implies insight into the assumptions and metaphors that shape our thinking. Metaphors can exert a dramatic effect on how an organization's mission is formulated and what sorts of plans we develop for achieving it. The best forms of knowledge sharing continually challenge such assumptions, and thereby foster the development of new, creative approaches.

When we teach medical students and residents, we should bear in mind the importance of knowledge sharing, focusing less on the recitation of information than the cultivation of creativity and collaboration. Wherever possible, learners should be challenged to tackle problems in small groups. Moreover, we should be evaluated not only as individuals but also as teams, a model adopted by most business schools decades ago. The emphasis should be on group work, teambuilding, and cultivating the skills necessary to function effectively as a team member. This requires educators to balance the traditional emphasis on individual competition with a new focus on group cooperation. Learners need to experience firsthand the difference in performance between a collection of individuals and a synergistic group, and gain some insight into how to transform the former into the latter.

A key distinction is that between information and knowledge. T. S. Eliot famously wrote, "Where is the wisdom we have lost in knowledge? Where is the knowledge we have lost in information?" Information is merely a tool, which may or may not be useful in the achievement of a particular objective. Knowledge, by contrast, represents the purposes for which we use information. What are we trying to do, and why? The use of new information technologies in education can open up access to information, yet over-reliance on technology often merely floods people with data. This in turn contributes to a self-defeating sense of inadequacy and confusion. Downloading data is not the same thing as fostering insight, and learners need to know the difference. We need to think of those we educate less as solitary data storage devices and more as collaborative investigators.

Knowledge is most fruitfully conceptualized not in mechanical terms but in biological terms. Knowledge sharing should be likened to sexual reproduction, in which genetic interchange permits the creation of new offspring who represent more than the mere sum of their parents. The goal is not to copy and transmit, but to recombine and even mutate. For example, new ideas are frequently produced when faculty members look at their work from the perspectives of other disciplines. Transdisciplinary and interdisciplinary perspectives help investigators to question unrecognized assumptions, consider novel approaches to solving problems, and develop new goals and outcomes measures.

Opportunities for synergy can be undermined by ineffective approaches to leadership and organization. When we confuse knowledge with information, we tend to suppose that all we need do to promote knowledge sharing is to put in place technological systems for the capture, storage, retrieval, and transmission of information. Such models promote the erroneous view that knowledge is an inert substance that can be transferred like any other supply, such as pencils and paper clips. In fact, however, it is difficult to divorce knowledge from the individuals who discover, synthesize, interpret, disseminate, and utilize it. We can send someone information, but we cannot send them knowledge.

In organizations dominated by authoritarian hierarchies, rigid command structures, and strong commitments to entrenched ranks and territories, knowledge sharing is likely to be inhibited. In such organizations, individuals define ourselves in large part by our ability to limit and control others' access to information. Free sharing of knowledge appears irrational because it undermines authority and competitive advantage. The more rapid the pace of change, however, the lower the probability that a few knowledge brokers at the top can formulate effective strategies. Moreover, treating members as though our duty were simply carrying out orders is likely to undermine our creativity and sense of commitment to the organization's success. This latter consideration is especially important in the case of physicians and scientists, who place a premium on professional autonomy.

Specialization and division of labor enable individuals to enhance the distinctiveness of our own perspectives and contributions. In an organization where people do not share what we know, each must know at least a little about many things, limiting understanding to a fairly superficial level. By contrast, a knowledge-sharing organization enables people to take full advantage of specialization, permitting each individual to understand more deeply a distinctive aspect of the organization's work. To enhance opportunities for such specialization, academic medical centers need to foster less competition and more interdependence. Opportunities for conversation and collaboration between disciplines should be cultivated. People need to appreciate that we are only as good as our colleagues and that by improving our colleagues' understanding, we are improving our own, as well.

To achieve such sharing, however, the organization needs to be permeated by a shared sense of mission. Incentive and reward systems that pit individuals or parts of an organization against one another can be self-defeating. So can lines of communication and authority that encourage individuals to think in purely local and self-interested modes. Leaders should be looking for regular opportunities to get people to plan in more global contexts, regarding our own contributions in terms of the whole organization. Every faculty member should be able to describe how our job fits into the overall mission of the organization, and why interacting with others is so vital in enabling everyone to do well. Status and rewards within the organization should hinge in part on each person's contributions to knowledge sharing. Specifically, departments need to develop a new kind of physician, one who freely shares ideas and expertise across the academic medical center.

Amid the frenetic pace of contemporary medicine, simply getting the members of a department together can prove a daunting challenge. Many organizations are so widely dispersed that people rarely see one another, and when they do, they are so preoccupied with their own immediate concerns that they have little time or interest in meaningful interchange. Occasions to think out loud, trade insights, and critique one another's ideas have been lost. If people are to cooperate fruitfully, we need face time, and leaders need to be deeply invested in ensuring that people are engaged in meaningful discussion on a regular basis. If people feel that we are being manipulated into something we do not want to do, a program of regular meetings may backfire, but so long as such meetings are appropriately organized and facilitated, good people will quickly realize that the benefits far outweigh the costs.

The best leaders excel at encouraging people to share what we know, not only with each other, but with our leaders, as well. A dictatorial style of leadership sets an example that discourages knowledge sharing, thereby limiting the knowledge of those in charge. People are less willing to share perspectives with an autocrat. Yet leaders need access to a variety of perspectives, in part because those who attempt to navigate with narrow or shallow outlooks typically fail. To facilitate such knowledge sharing, the leader needs to be regarded more as a colleague than a boss, someone with whom people can talk frankly without fear of betrayal or punishment. Leaders should think of themselves as catalysts in a chemical reaction. Without them, little would happen. Operating alone, however, they are incapable of producing anything.

The quality of everything physicians do – patient care, education, research, and service – hinges on the sharing of knowledge. The mindset that knowledge is a tangible good and its pursuit a zero-sum game represents a profoundly debilitating misconception. Departments will make themselves stronger by promoting knowledge sharing among members, schools will make themselves stronger by promoting knowledge sharing across departments, and medicine will make itself stronger by promoting knowledge sharing among schools. Leaders should not expect to achieve a technological fix – faster and wider data sharing – for what is fundamentally a sociological problem – getting people talking with one another. At every level of academic medicine, the guiding ideal should be that of the true university. The target is not a jumble of intellectual fiefdoms, each jealously guarding its precious cache of information, but a dynamic community that thrives on the sharing of knowledge.

Chapter 8
Searching for a Leader

The search for leaders is one of the most important challenges facing medical practices and healthcare organizations. When a search is successful and the right person lands in the right job, the organization may continue to reap benefits for years, even decades. Yet some searches fail, and the resultant suffering can prove equally enduring. Because an outstanding leader affords an organization so many benefits, while a terrible leader exacts a high price, it is vital that physicians and health professionals devote substantial attention to the recruitment and selection of leaders.

Two of the greatest dangers in the search for a leader are ignorance and apathy. Preoccupied by other demands, some organizations neglect the process. They assume that past momentum will carry the organization forward, no matter who is in charge. Yet even great organizations can be undone by poor leadership. The people whose lives will be most affected by the choice of leader have the greatest vested interest in ensuring that the organization gets the best person for the job.

One relatively neglected issue is retention of good leaders. Many leaders receive only one kind of appraisal – complaints. Leaders hear about problems in the organization on a daily basis, but when things work well, words of praise are sparse. No one realizes that leaders have their own doubts and insecurities, and need occasional words of encouragement just like everyone else. Leaders, too, need to learn, grow, and find fulfillment in work. We forget how lonely the leader's job can

R.B. Gunderman, *Leadership in Healthcare*,
DOI 10.1007/978-1-84800-943-1_8,
© Springer-Verlag London Limited 2009

be. One of the most important contributions each of us can make to the welfare of our organizations is to provide appreciative performance appraisals to leaders who deserve them. This is a contribution that each one of us is capable of making.

It is important that responsible people take the search for leaders seriously. If the search is a perfunctory one that no one really believes in, the search itself – regardless its outcome – will take a toll on organizational morale. In academic organizations, conducting a regional or national search is preferable to promptly selecting an internal candidate. This approach shows that the organization cares about its leadership and means to find the best candidate. It also provides candidates and members of the organization an opportunity to develop their own visions for the future of the organization. What alternative courses could the organization pursue, and what are the advantages and disadvantages of each?

People who find the effort involved in a leadership search daunting need only consider the costs of failure. Uncivil leaders tend to offend people and squander opportunities for learning, collaboration, and growth. Arrogant leaders tend to communicate badly and act arbitrarily, damaging morale throughout the organization. Insecure leaders tend to be distrustful, and their failure to share responsibility squelches others' development as leaders. Isolated leaders tend to undermine unity by adopting policies that pit different groups against one another. Socially inept leaders tend to compromise recruiting efforts. In the worst-case scenario, a leader's duplicity may cast a pall of suspicion over an entire organization.

Leadership transitions should be seen as natural stages in the life of every organization. The question is not if they will occur, but how well. When a transition is planned in advance, it is possible to appoint a successor before the departing leader steps down, and the two can work together to ensure a smooth transition. Unexpected vacancies are bound to arise from time to time, and in some cases, months or even years may elapse before a successor can be appointed. Interim periods between leaders can delay important choices, create a general atmosphere of indecision, inhibit recruiting, and leave the organization vulnerable to others who may not have its best interests at heart. People may begin to look for greener pastures elsewhere, creating additional vacancies. As people leave, those who remain may feel increasingly overworked and discouraged, contributing to a vicious spiral of departures and discontent. As those who remain find it harder and harder just to keep up, other missions may suffer, making the organization less attractive to top prospects.

Why do leaders leave? One problem is a mismatch between responsibility and authority. Some leaders are held responsible for everything that goes wrong, yet lack the means to prevent problems and enhance performance. To prevent this sort of problem, we need to trust our leaders and give them the authority and tools they need to do their jobs. Another problem is the failure of some leaders to develop lieutenants with whom they can share responsibility. Particularly in large organizations, where there is a great deal of work to be done, such governance structures can be crucial to a leader's effectiveness and longevity. A third difficulty is the frequently stunted intellectual life of leaders. If academic organizations are doing their jobs, they will appoint leaders with strong academic credentials, whose vision extend beyond a single facet of the mission, such as clinical service. Yet if we allow clinical operations to consume all of leaders' time and energy, the loss of other interests and abilities may cause their sense of fulfillment to wane.

The search for a leader should prompt a serious examination of the organization, not just who is going to lead it. Important questions need to be asked, by both the organization itself and the candidates who interview for the position. Does the organization have a clear picture of its own mission? How effectively has it been able to achieve it? What resources are available to pursue its goals? What additional resources are needed, and is the institution prepared to commit them? What are the organization's most important internal weaknesses? Will the leader have the authority and tools necessary to redress them? What external challenges face the organization, and what plans are in place to meet them? Are there any skeletons in the closet that a prospective leader should be informed about?

What is the culture of the organization, in terms of its commitment to excellence, approaches to communication and problem solving, and past leadership styles? How great a challenge would it be to lead this organization? Is the institution prepared to invest in the leader's development as a manager and a leader, and what opportunities would it make available? What is the level of commitment of other leaders to the health of the organization, and what role does the organization play regarding their own opportunities for success? One useful technique for getting to know an organization is a so-called SWOT analysis (strengths, weaknesses, opportunities, threats), which provides valuable insight into what leadership attributes might matter most.

When a candidate interviews for a leadership position, it is vital that he or she quickly adopt a perspective that places the long-term interests of the organization foremost. In the first place, an effective search and screen committee should quickly weed out candidates whose primary focus is on their own personal success. More importantly, a transition in leadership presents an important opportunity for the organization to secure greater support from parent organizations such as hospitals and medical schools. Rather than feeling flattered at being considered for the position, serious candidates should function as the organization's advocate, basing their negotiating position on a sober assessment of the organization's needs and local resources to meet them. Major bargaining points might include new equipment, more space, new or renovated facilities, supplementation of faculty salaries, expansion of educational programs, more representation in key policy-making forums, a larger discretionary fund for the leader, a serious commitment to the ongoing education of organizational leadership, and a greater role for the organization in major fundraising campaigns, among many other possibilities.

No health professional should seriously consider assuming leadership responsibility before making an earnest commitment to the flourishing of the organization. In most cases, recruitment represents one of the best opportunities a prospective leader will ever enjoy to bargain for the means to success. When a candidate leaps immediately at a leadership position, the organization misses out on this opportunity, and a good search committee should recognize such conduct as a sign of weakness that will almost certainly redound to the organization's detriment.

What should organizations seek in a prospective leader? Key questions must be addressed. Is the candidate a person of integrity? Is the candidate an autocrat or a team builder? Is the candidate the type of leader who tends to act independently and shoot from the hip, or someone who consults with others before making important decisions? Is the candidate good with people, someone others look up to and feel comfortable talking with? Will the candidate promote two-way communication throughout the organization, enabling everyone to make better-informed choices? Is the candidate patient, someone who can resist the "tyranny of the annual report" and do what longer-term interests require? Is he or she gifted with common sense, the ability to see through what fogs the judgment of others? Is the candidate capable of making tough decisions and delivering bad news? Will the candidate be able to cope with adversity, to maintain a clear sense of purpose amid an atmosphere of crisis, and to remain focused and energetic when others might throw in the towel?

Is the candidate able to articulate a clear mission for the organization and the role he or she would play in achieving it? How well does the candidate understand the organization and the larger institution and healthcare environment in which it is situated? How would the candidate respond to real or even hypothetical challenges? What mistakes has the candidate made in the past, how did he or she respond to them, and what lessons were learned? How much insight does the candidate display into his or her strengths and weaknesses as a leader? Is the candidate a successful health professional who will be respected by others, both locally and nationally? Does he or she bring a proven track record as a researcher, educator, or administrator? Or does the candidate view this leadership post as a way to jumpstart a sagging career?

A good leader must be prepared to deal with personnel issues that might seem trivial to an outside observer but crucial to the people involved. Many of these issues, and perhaps 90% of what the leader does, generate as much frustration as fulfillment. Yet leaders must be able to see past responsibilities that are not intrinsically rewarding and derive satisfaction from the 10% of activities that are truly challenging and enjoyable. Dealing with complex issues and problems is part of the leader's mission, and he or she must earnestly engage such problems, despite their lack of intrinsic fascination. In this respect, a good leader needs to be not only unselfish but also optimistic and capable of fostering a sense of optimism in others.

The measure of successful leaders is not how famous they have become, but how well their organizations have fared under their leadership. Great leaders focus less on their own achievement than on the achievements of the organizations they lead. They are able to subordinate their own personal ambitions to these larger goals. The chief responsibility of good leaders is not to propel themselves to national prominence, but to find satisfaction through the success of others. What the leader does is less important than what the leader enables others to do, and many new leaders have failed precisely because they could not make the transition from working for themselves to working on behalf of others.

The leader's mission is to recruit and retain good people, to nurture the abilities of others, and to recognize and reward excellence. For this reason, very high achievers do not necessarily make the best leaders. Their need for personal achievement may override their commitment to the best interests of the organization. In most cases, a good leader more resembles the coach of a successful sports team than a monarchical ruler. To determine whether a candidate genuinely seeks to serve, a selection committee should carefully seek out evidence of service, past coaching and mentoring, and a commitment to meeting the needs and promoting the interests of others.

Selection committees should assure themselves that candidates understand their mission. Key questions should be posed. How much time does the candidate believe would be required to excel? What other professional pursuits, such as research, education, or clinical work, would the candidate propose to continue? Does the candidate have major personal commitments, and how would he or she balance personal life and leadership? For the right person, a leadership position opens up new possibilities for professional fulfillment. For the wrong person, however, leadership can be a painful experience, at best merely interrupting an otherwise successful career.

An individual who assumes a leadership post must work hard to find ways to continue to thrive personally and professionally in the midst of the many demands it entails. While no two leaders are exactly alike, the best ones share certain leadership traits in common, including high personal integrity, strong skills in strategic planning and communication, a deep commitment to the academic missions that define the future of the field, and a willingness to subordinate the pursuit of their own achievement to that of their colleagues, their department, their institution, and their profession.

The search for leadership is not a purely external one. Just as we need to look around for effective leaders, so we need to look within ourselves to locate and develop our own leadership capabilities. Some of the most important internal barriers to leadership development are our habits of thought and feeling. Many of us have the potential to make important contributions, but we fail to realize it because these habits hold us back. If we can learn to identify and redress them, we can free ourselves up to do a better job as leaders. These same lessons can help us to nurture colleagues' leadership potential.

***

How can we respond more effectively to such common but debilitating sentiments as despair, anxiety, and rage? Cognitive therapy is a psychological approach developed in the 1950s and 1960s by two important American psychologists, Albert Ellis and Aaron Beck. It challenged the prevailing psychoanalytic view that immutable biological drives and repressed fears and conflicts necessarily dominate our lives. Cognitive therapists argue that if we focus rationally on our immediate feelings and perceptions we can enhance our responses to the events of our lives.

Ellis developed what he called the A–B–C model for describing the relationship between our experiences and our reactions. By exploring our lives in terms of this framework, we can identify and modify patterns of thought that prevent us from performing at our best and from enjoying life to the fullest possible extent. He called these constraining patterns of thought "irrational beliefs," although "distortions" might be a better term.

A stands for "activating event." Activating events are simply the statements, actions, and situations we encounter on a daily basis. There are numerous examples. A colleague points out a clinical error. A colleague asks for help in completing a research project. A colleague complains about some aspect of the work environment, such as the poor quality of the support staff or the unfair administrative policies. Of course, activating events need not be passive and can also be actions we take ourselves. For example, failing to complete a project on schedule is also an activating event. In Ellis's framework, it is important to consider activating events as objectively as possible, omitting our own reactions to them.

B stands for "belief." In this phase, we consider what the event means to us. To some degree, the separation of events from beliefs is artificial because our perceptions of events are always colored by our beliefs about them. When a layperson and a physician look at a chest radiograph, they see quite different things, even though the photons striking their retinas convey identical sensory data. There is no completely objective, "belief-free" perspective from which any of us can view the world. Nevertheless, our beliefs affect how we interpret events, and different beliefs may lead to radically different interpretations. For example, why would a colleague draw attention to an error? Is it to help us perform better or just one more attempt to "bring us down?"

A cinematic drama that captures the importance of belief is Akira Kurosawa's "Rashamon" (1950), one of the greatest films ever made (Fig. 8.1). Set in eleventh century Japan, it tells the story of a forest encounter between a bandit, a samurai, and the samurai's beautiful young wife. The samurai winds up

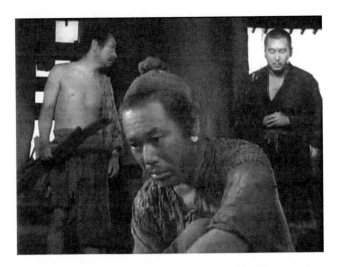

Fig. 8.1 Takashi Shimura as the woodcutter in Akira Kurosawa's cinematic masterpiece, *Rashomon* (1950). The story's characters offer radically different accounts of a dramatic event, leaving viewers to determine which one, if any, is true

dead, the woman is found hiding in a temple, and the police apprehend the bandit with the dead man's possessions. Each of these characters, as well as a passing woodsman, offers radically different accounts of what transpired. From one point of view, it seems that the bandit lusted after the woman, killed her husband, and raped her. From another point of view, it seems that the jealous samurai attacked the bandit and was killed in self-defense. From a third point of view, it seems that the liaison between the bandit and the woman was consensual, and the latter killed her husband to escape a miserable marriage. As we weigh these different perspectives, the film challenges us to examine our own beliefs.

C refers to "consequent emotion." How do we feel about what happened? Ellis realized that belief powerfully affects our feelings. If we interpret a colleague's actions as an attempt to help us perform better, then our consequent emotion will be gratitude. On the other hand, if we see the situation as an attempt to make us look bad, then our reaction may be anger, even a thirst for revenge. One of the most important insights of cognitive therapy is the realization that our interpretations, and more importantly, our patterns of interpretation, are usually not set in stone. Over time, we can actually change the stereotypical patterns by which we react to the world around us. In other words, changing the way we think (interpret events) can change the way we feel and even how we are capable of responding.

Aaron Beck described a number of common irrational beliefs or distortions that may cloud our thinking. By recognizing and then working on characteristic psychological distortions, Beck argued, we can think our way out of many otherwise depressing, nerve-racking, or enraging situations. Among these, distortions are "catastrophizing," minimizing, dichotomous thinking, emotional reasoning, fortune telling, labeling, mind reading, over-generalization, and personalization. Do we recognize ourselves and our organizations in some of these descriptions? What can we do to overcome them?

People who engage in catastrophizing tend to overestimate the importance of events. Psychoanalysts often interpreted cigars and umbrellas in phallic terms, but Freud himself said that "Sometimes a cigar is just a cigar." Casual remarks and actions may sometimes reveal far more than we think, but in many cases they do not necessarily bear far-reaching implications. Yet some of us tend to seize on little things and magnify their importance beyond what an objective observer would infer. We see criticisms and insults where none were intended, or magnify tiny scratches into mortal wounds. Making a mountain out of a mole hill can lead to many problems for leaders, including distrust. Others may come to believe that we are unable to see events in their true proportion.

Minimizing is a similar problem, oriented in the opposite direction. Minimizing is typical of ungrateful people, who do not recognize the extent to which others are genuinely trying to help them. They regard genuine kindnesses as expressions of mere etiquette, superficial and inconsequential. To say that every event in life is not a crisis does not compel us to say that no event in life is truly important. The mark of a wise person is not the conviction that all events are either monumental or trivial, but an appropriate assessment of the significance of each. One of the keys to leading a happy and productive life and helping others to do the same is to distinguish appropriately between the two.

Dichotomous thinking means recognizing and choosing between just two alternatives when other better options are available. For example, a department chair may feel that the hospital is not responding appropriately to capital equipment requests. A dichotomous reaction would be to deliver an ultimatum: "Either we get the equipment we need, or we leave the hospital." In fact, however, many more options may be available. For example, the two organizations might work together to develop a creative solution, such as a lease, which enables the hospital to expend less capital yet provide the department the equipment it needs.

Emotional reasoning and fortune telling are rampant among pessimists. Some people see a glass as half full, others see it as half empty. While both statements are true, one embodies a more optimistic outlook than the other. In general, optimism is more conducive to hope and action. Emotional reasoning is dangerous because we may interpret our feeling of dread or despair as inherently embedded in the situation we confront, when in fact someone else might see great opportunity among the challenges. Mistakes and defeats may be inevitable parts of life, but there is no need to treat every challenge as merely another opportunity to fail. Great leaders are not defined by the ability to realize before everyone else that a situation is hopeless. Quite the contrary, great leaders see cause for hope where others despair.

Labeling occurs when we make broad inferences about a person's character based on a single statement or action. For example, the first time we meet a new colleague, we may draw firm conclusions, even though subsequent events contradict them. At their worst, labelers tend to categorize people according to such terms as "idiot" or "loser." Yet if we really believe that our characters are malleable and that each of us is capable of becoming an even better person, then we should remain open to the possibility of reform and even redemption. People who tend to make hasty judgments can become more deliberate. People who have difficulty making choices can become more decisive. People who tend to see the worst in others can learn to be more trusting and hopeful.

Mind readers believe that they understand exactly what people are thinking and feeling based on their actions. To deny that we can infer intentions based on actions would be absurd. Yet some of us tend to overestimate our abilities in this regard. Major conflicts and missed opportunities result when we fundamentally misunderstand who others are and what they are about. Instead of supposing that we can read other people's minds, we need to take the time to talk with them. We need to find out how they see events, what they are trying to accomplish, and who they really are. Taking time for such conversations not only enhances our understanding but also gives us a chance to show others that we care about them.

Overgeneralization occurs when we take one event as proof of a pattern that we see in a series of events. For example, if a colleague makes a careless error, we might interpret every error as carelessness, when in fact more important systematic sources are responsible that have nothing to do with the colleague. What seems like carelessness may reflect a defective information system or faulty organizational habits of communication. Overgeneralizing can be attractive, because it saves mental effort. Rather than reflect on each instance in its own right, we can simply attribute all of them to a single cause. Yet by failing to reexamine situations, we needlessly consign ourselves to underperformance and poor relationships. Before condemning others, we should look more deeply, and then look again.

Personalization occurs when our preferred response to adverse outcomes is to look for someone to blame. This impulse comports with our society's growing litigiousness, which recasts suffering as a harm calling for civil remedies. Adverse outcomes are not necessarily the fault of any single person or group of people. Instead of reflexively blaming someone, we should inquire more deeply to identify the real sources of error. Conversely, good outcomes are not necessarily the result of any single person's efforts, and we need to be prepared to apportion praise and appreciation more widely.

Cognitive therapy is important because it moves our emotions and reactions from the domain of things that merely happen to us to the domain of things over which we exert influence. Before we despair or become enraged at events, we would do well to ponder these common psychological pitfalls. By employing the techniques of cognitive therapy, we can search for alternative perspectives that enhance performance and promote a greater degree of personal and professional fulfillment.

***

One of the most important characteristics of effective leaders is the ability to learn from error. To secure good leaders, our organizations need to do a better job of cultivating this ability. Learning from errors requires a different kind of preparation than most physicians received during professional education. It does not mean memorizing the answers to questions, solving problems, or developing proficiency at new technical skills. Instead it involves critically inspecting our daily work and practice systems, seeking ways to improve them as opportunities arise. In essence, we need to be more reflective and even skeptical about the way we do things, and think creatively about how we could do better.

To enhance our capacity to learn from error, we need to do three things. First, we need to make a commitment to raise our level of performance. So long as we regard the status quo as sufficient, improvement is unlikely. Second, we need to see errors as opportunities. They are not diseases that we need to eradicate, but symptoms of flawed structures and processes that we can improve. When we see errors as opportunities, they cease to be something to hide and become some of our favorite things to explore. Third, we need to recognize the barriers to openness that beset many healthcare organizations. By identifying and deepening our understanding of these barriers, we can enhance learning from error and raise our level of performance.

One important barrier to openness is the sense of shame we feel when others see our errors. By nature, most physicians like to be right. Even more, we hate to be wrong. We naturally fear that if others see our mistakes, they will think less of us. Patients may go elsewhere for care. Colleagues may send their patients to other physicians or facilities. Supervisors may overlook us in decisions about hiring, promotion, and tenure. If others see us as error prone, perhaps even merely fallible, we may not achieve the level of respect we aspire to.

This excessive sense of shame is one of the most corrosive attitudes in contemporary healthcare organizations, which leads us to keep errors (learning opportunities) under raps. We begin by hiding mistakes from others, but we end up hiding them from ourselves. When this happens, we deprive ourselves and our organizations of one of our most valuable resources. We become so wrapped up in preserving the illusion of our own infallibility that we no longer see errors for what they are and forego the opportunity for improvement they offer. In effect, we allow pride to subvert our curiosity and aspiration for excellence.

The better justification for pride in work is not infallibility but a deep commitment to learning. To create a learning culture, we need to inspire a sense of optimism and trust. We need to convince ourselves and others that mistakes are not lethal and that we can not only survive them but also grow from them. Moreover, we need to show everyone that we will treat errors not as occasions for mean spiritedness and invective but as opportunities to enhance performance. When we see mistakes as symptoms of more fundamental problems, we begin to place less emphasis on who made them and focus more on what they tell us about our organizational systems. For example, an error traceable to a breakdown in communication may tell us less about the communicators than about the systems through which we share our knowledge, perspectives, and experiences.

If the search for scapegoats is so counterproductive, why is it so popular? The blame game is attractive for a number of reasons. First, our system of medical education tends to foster the view that every error is traceable to an individual. Throughout our training, every exam we take has right and wrong answers. We treat incorrect answers as the fault of the examinee, not the fault of the educational system. Second, our preoccupation with malpractice fosters the view that every adverse outcome stems from negligence. If everyone were doing their job properly, we seem to suppose, how could errors occur? Third, finding someone to blame gives us an outlet for tension, guilt, and even anger associated with error. By heaping blame on someone else, we think we can lighten our own loads. Such blame is hazardous, because it drives errors deep underground where they cannot be seen and learned from.

Most of us are attracted to the ideals of autonomy and independence. It is comforting to think that everything depends on our dedication and expertise. It implies that when things go well, we deserve the credit. Yet such attitudes can undermine a culture of information sharing and collective learning. Instead of focusing on the decisions of individual practitioners, we can do better by defining patterns of practice conducive to collective excellence. Health care is less an individual sport than a team sport, and we need to focus more on the long-term performance of organizations and less on the short-term performance of individuals. To reduce errors and improve performance, we need to improve our systems more than we need to find individuals to blame.

What can we do to mitigate the sense of shame that inhibits the open exploration of error? First, by promoting a culture that prizes learning from errors, we can eliminate the debilitating fear that we are the only ones making mistakes. Everyone makes mistakes, and anyone who greets this assertion with incredulity reveals ignorance, not infallibility. Second, we need to make it clear to everyone that recognizing and sharing errors will not meet with reprisals. This is particularly important when the mistakes in question are being made by people in positions of authority. Another barrier to learning from errors is very wide dispersion of responsibility throughout an organization. If it is not clear who is responsible for different organizational missions, then it becomes too easy to blame others when things go wrong. Every leader should help to define who is responsible for detecting, investigating, and preventing errors.

Being open about errors makes sense only if the organization is truly committed to doing something about them. This means developing and improving systems for detecting, sharing, and responding to errors. Simply maintaining a list of things that have gone wrong offers little opportunity to make things better. What procedures are in place for identifying risks? What avenues are available for sharing lessons learned? Who is accountable for ensuring that changes are made? Do people ever meet to discuss the answers to these questions? Are such opportunities regular items on meeting agendas, and do people genuinely prize the opportunity to learn from each other? If nothing ever happens to improve matters, people will lose their faith in the process.

We can devise all manner of professional, civil, and even criminal penalties to discourage mistakes. We can implement any number of financial, professional, and social rewards for those who avoid them. What we most need, however, is a paradigm shift in the way we think about error. Centuries ago, the profession of medicine operated according to a paradigm that highly prize blood letting. So long as it did so, therapeutic results remained deeply constrained. So long as we operate in a paradigm that regards error as a disease of the error prone, our excellence will be stunted. We need a paradigm shift in the way we think about error, one that recognizes errors as valuable insights into the systems we work by.

Chapter 9
Developing Leaders

Future leaders need to understand human psychology. Key leadership activities such as communication, motivation, team building, and planning all draw on our understanding of other people. Before we can help colleagues to perform at their best, we need to understand how they think and feel, especially about the major projects that characterize their lives. This means getting to know each person individually, but it also means understanding the universal developmental tasks that each of us faces as we go through life. By enhancing our understanding of developmental psychology, we can prepare ourselves to help colleagues negotiate these transitions successfully and perform at their best.

One of the most influential developmental psychologists of the twentieth century was Erik Erikson (Fig. 9.1). Erikson was born in 1902 in Germany of Danish parents. Though tall, blond, and blue-eyed, Erikson was raised a Jew by his mother and stepfather. He was mocked in religious school for his Nordic appearance and in grammar school for his religion, which may help to explain his life-long interest in identity. In 1933, Erikson emigrated to the United States, where he became the first child psychoanalyst in Boston. He held faculty positions at Harvard, Yale, and the University of California at Berkeley. Despite his immense influence on the field of psychology, Erickson earned no degree beyond a high school diploma.

Erikson is perhaps best known for his eight-stage theory of psychosocial development, which centers around stereotypical

R.B. Gunderman, *Leadership in Healthcare*,
DOI 10.1007/978-1-84800-943-1_9,
© Springer-Verlag London Limited 2009

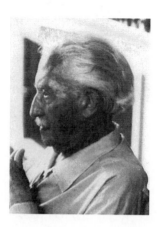

Fig. 9.1 Erik Erikson (1902–1994), one of the twentieth century's foremost developmental psychologists, though he never earned a degree beyond a high school diploma. He described eight life-stage virtues, which may be acquired in the following order: hope, will, purpose, competence, fidelity, love, caring, and wisdom

life problems or challenges that confront each person over the course of a lifetime. He believed that we can achieve coherent identity only by mastering these developmental challenges. He thought that these stages occur in sequence from childhood through adulthood, but we may confront these issues again and again as our lives unfold.

Before considering the light Erikson's theory sheds on leadership, several points need to be highlighted. First, each of us negotiates these stages with greater or lesser degrees of success. Many of us return to certain issues during our life, because they have not been successfully resolved. Second, if we have failed to work out some of these issues, we may engage in counterproductive conduct that alienates others and compromises our effectiveness. Third, in contrast to Freud's developmental theories, we are not set in our ways when we leave adolescence, and each of us has the opportunity to continue to develop throughout our lives. Finally, one of the common threads running through each of Erikson's stages is the ongoing tension between affiliation and connectedness, on the one hand, and autonomy and independence, on the other. Following is an examination of six of Erickson's eight stages, with a discussion of how each might apply in healthcare leadership.

The first developmental stage is trust versus mistrust. Members of any organization need to be able to trust its leaders. When we join a new department, we are uncertain how things work. We seek opportunities to become integrated and feel that we are part of the group. While we are developing our own sense of competence in the new organization, we need others whom we can rely on to look out for us and help us through the new challenges we face. If people in the organization, particularly new members, believe that leaders are aloof and mysterious or operate capriciously, this trust will be difficult to establish. Likewise, if leadership positions are unfilled, or there is rapid turnover, people will find it difficult to feel secure and comfortable in the organization. A lack of trust, in turn, makes it difficult to function as loyal and committed members of the team. If future healthcare leaders are to perform at our best, we must become adept at building and sustaining trust among patients, colleagues, and the community.

In today's rapidly changing healthcare environment, leaders also need to foster innovation and a willingness to take risks. A top–down model of leadership in which everyone follows one person's direction is untenable, because it fails to take advantage of the insights and perspectives of too many capable people in the organization. A more participative model of leadership enables the organization to take advantage of a variety of perspectives, by promoting better informed choices at the top and by enabling colleagues to react promptly to new challenges and opportunities on the "front lines." For this to happen, however, we must believe that our leaders value our contributions, even those over which there may be disagreement. We also need to feel that we can count on leaders to support us, so long as we are trying to do what we think is best for the organization and those it serves. We need encouragement to try out new things, knowing that mistakes will inevitably occur. If we are criticized every time we attempt to think for ourselves, and if conformity becomes the organization's highest value, then creativity will be squelched.

Erikson thought that people encounter identity crises at multiple points in life. In the course of becoming a physician, there are transitions from medical student to resident, from junior resident to senior resident, from resident to fellow, and from fellow to attending physician. At each transition, we face issues of incompetence versus mastery, disinterest versus interest, and outsider versus colleague. Courses and examinations do not merely transmit information and weed out individuals who do not meet minimum thresholds. They also help people negotiate these transitions. Doing so successfully enables us to believe that we have sufficiently mastered a body of knowledge and skills, determined what most interests us, and established ourselves as legitimate members of a professional group. One of our greatest burdens is uncertainty. We are confronted by questions: What am I supposed to be doing? Am I doing it? Do other people think I am doing well? By helping to establish clear performance expectations and providing constructive criticism, leaders can help colleagues clarify identity and aspirations.

Role models play a crucial role in medical leadership. They need not be perfect, but they need to be people we can look up to and trust. They help us define what we are most passionately committed to. They are dedicated not so much to impressing their personality on everyone else, but to enabling others to redress weaknesses and develop strengths. They help us develop a sense of who we are, as professionals and as human beings, a self-concept that helps to anchor us in tumultuous times.

If we fail to develop a clear sense of who we are, we are likely to perform poorly not only as leaders but also as followers and teammates. Erikson described several difficulties to which such people are predisposed. What he called role diffusion makes it difficult to discern what really matters, which in turn makes it difficult to work with passion. Such people are easily led astray, and this lack of a strong "compass" may cause others to stray as well. Such people may develop role foreclosure, adopting someone else's ideas without thinking things through personally. It may require years or even decades to discern that we have followed the wrong path, and by that point, it may be very difficult to get back on track. Unfortunately, many healthcare organizations are organized so that such discussions rarely take place. A leader's mission is to help us honestly confront the identity questions we face and give them the consideration they deserve.

Many of us come to work out of a need for affiliation and the desire to develop and sustain colleagiality. We need to believe that we and our colleagues are real people with real lives, not just interchangeable cogs in a machine. We need to know that we can share our lives, look out for one another, and rejoice and commiserate together. As healthcare organizations become busier, larger, and more complex, a sense of community becomes harder and harder to sustain. To counteract this centrifugal tendency, leaders need to find opportunities to bring people together, both literally and figuratively. Regular conferences, lunches, and holiday parties in which everyone participates are important, especially in larger organizations. In a healthy organization, people talk and act like members of the same team, with respect and even affection for colleagues.

Early in our careers, many physicians function more as takers than givers. We are consumers of knowledge, consumers of advice, and consumers of career development resources. With time, however, we can make a transition to a generative role, in which we are not only taking but also giving back. It is more fulfilling to give, to help others develop their insights and abilities, than to receive. As long as we are confined to the role of recipient, we will find it difficult to lead others, to take responsibility for the policies and practices, and to invest in the organization's growth and development. Generative people see our lives not as a series of snapshots but as a motion picture, one that continues even after we are gone. We look beyond the expediency of the moment to the interests of those who will follow in our footsteps and blaze new trails in years to come. We aim to invest in the future of departments, hospitals, and universities, contributing not only money but also time and attention to building a better world. We aspire not only to make our own stars shine more brightly but those of others, too. Such people represent the lifeblood of every organization.

People who do not achieve an outlook of generativity tend to stagnate. We live for ourselves and contribute little to others, who quickly sense that we are interested only in ourselves. The quality of our relationships suffers. Less well liked than others, our ability to collaborate and be a meaningful part of teams is compromised. This can become a vicious cycle, in which lack of generativity breeds isolation, which in turn breeds increasing stagnation. Good leaders look for ways to encourage colleagues to work toward ends greater than ourselves. Opportunities include chairing a fund-raiser, serving on an education committee, taking an active role in mentoring junior colleagues, or becoming involved in community service. One of the best opportunities is education, which focuses our attention on the needs of learners and helps us to keep learning. Organizations need to recognize and praise service activities and provide role models for the next generation of healthcare leaders.

Retirement is a risk-laden endeavor. Our ability to contribute is not exhausted just because we reach the age of 65 or 70. It is unreasonable to think that people who have worked throughout our adult lives will suddenly find fulfillment in a state of idleness, with nothing to focus on except our own amusement. As we age, we lose some of our energy and stamina, but few suffer a sudden collapse that renders us unable to work. One of the cruelest insults is to tell someone they can no longer contribute. Senior colleagues may be unable to produce at their former pace. Yet many can draw on years of experience and storehouses of wisdom that younger, more energetic colleagues may lack. We should be looking for ways to keep senior colleagues engaged in the profession.

People who fail to find opportunities to contribute meaningfully to others may even find ourselves in a state of despair. When we stagnate, we tend to become disillusioned, even bitter. We take out our frustrations on others, spending much of our time complaining and sowing the seeds of discontent. To prevent such outcomes, leaders need to be on the lookout for signs of stagnation and provide opportunities for colleagues to continue to be challenged and to grow throughout our careers. There is simply no point at which physicians and other health professionals can claim to know all that we will need to know.

Few physician leaders are likely to become experts in psychology, but it is vital that every physician, and especially every physician leader, be an avid student. Our perceptions of others' motivations and behaviors deeply shape our attempts at collaboration, and an incomplete or inaccurate understanding can wreak considerable harm. No matter how clinically knowledgeable or skilled we may be, if we do not understand what makes others tick, we will remain forever out of sync. A few gifted future leaders may be able to compensate for deficiencies in this area through instinct and intuition, but for the rest of us, the study of psychology is both necessary and fascinating.

***

To thrive, health care requires a number of important resources. These include the physical plants of our hospitals and outpatient facilities, capital equipment such as CT scanners and hospital information systems, supplies including tongue depressors and catheters, personnel such as clerical staff and housekeepers, and the knowledge and skills of physicians and other healthcare professionals. Yet missing from this list is another crucial resource that tends to receive less than its due. Ironically, it is one on which the future of our field depends to a growing extent. This resource is intellectual community.

When I took my first faculty job a decade ago, it was not uncommon to see five or more faculty members at our department's daily resident education conference. Now there is just one – the person giving the conference. When I first arrived, department members gathered for a well-attended faculty lunch once every 2 weeks. These days such large numbers do not gather more than several times each year. When I first arrived, I knew all the members of my department. Now there are colleagues that I have not seen in years, and some that I have never met.

The reasons for this erosion are numerous. Physicians are working harder and harder for longer and longer hours, which makes taking time out for a meeting an increasingly dear sacrifice. We are now more widely dispersed than we used to be, which means that we see one another less frequently and makes travel to a common meeting site more problematic. It has become more difficult for us to leave the point of care. Moreover, new information technology is making face-to-face contact with physicians, other health professionals, and even patients a rarer phenomenon. There is another reason for the decline of community, one that should arouse concern among physician leaders: a serious underestimation of the importance of intellectual community. If someone steals our trash, we do not express much concern. After all, we were prepared to discard it anyway. I fear that some of us regard the decline of intellectual community in medical departments and healthcare organizations with a similar level of indifference.

What is intellectual community? The word intellect is derived from the past participle of the Latin verb *intelligere* which means "to perceive." *Intelligere* in turn derives from the roots *inter-* meaning "between," and *legere*, "to choose." Hence intellect pertains to our capacity to recognize and choose between alternative explanations and courses of action. Community derives from the Latin *communitatis*, meaning "fellowship," from a root meaning "shared." What is our level of fellowship and shared understanding, and how well have we prepared our organizations to make the best choices? Intellectual community is vital. A Carnegie Foundation report, *The Formation of Scholars*, sheds considerable light on this subject. Intellectual community encompasses many of the crucial issues on which a discipline's future research and teaching depend. These include questions such as these: In this organization, how do people share ideas? How highly is teaching esteemed? How do medical students, residents, and fellows engage with faculty? How do we handle errors and failures? To what degree are people encouraged to raise questions and develop new creative approaches? How effectively do members of the department stay connected to the wider field?

If we ignore intellectual community, the quality of questions we pose, the answers we arrive at, and the effectiveness with which we share knowledge will all suffer. It is not just that the field of medicine will suffer. Individual departments will suffer, as well. When it comes to attracting and retaining the best medical students, residents, fellows, and faculty members, departments with little sense of intellectual community will be at a competitive disadvantage. They will become less engaging and rewarding places to work, precisely because people in them focus all their attention on getting the clinical work done. What is the level of intellectual engagement in our organizations? Is it high or low? Are people thinking about and discussing the key questions that will define the future of the field? Or have we given up, because we have too much work to do? While there is no doubt that a relatively small number of elite academic institutions will continue to play a very important role in these domains, it is deleterious for medicine if other educational institutions simply default on this responsibility because others are tending to it.

How often do we express a shared vision of how to help today's learners become tomorrow's leading teachers, researchers, and clinicians? How often do learners encounter rigorous intellectual debate? If all our disagreements are personal, or if disagreements are simply swept under the carpet, how will learners hone their skills in critical thinking and civil intellectual interchange? What level of diversity do learners encounter? Do people bring a range of different ideas and perspectives to work? As what we have come to call clinical productivity fills our field of view, what priority are we assigning to our ability to think? How often do we provide ourselves with room – spatial, temporal, and intellectual – in which to try out new ideas? What are we doing to counteract our own heavy bias toward positive results, encouraging everyone to talk about ideas and approaches that failed? We can learn a lot more from one another by discussing our setbacks than by simply patting one another on the back, as though no one ever makes a mistake.

To what degree are faculty members engaged in discussions about what we teach, how it ought to be taught, and how we evaluate learners? How often are members of the department engaged in interdepartmental conferences, and to what extent are learners participating in such forums? It is bad enough if they are not active participants, but even worse if they are not even present. What do researchers and teachers know about one another's approaches? Such knowledge can provide a rich stimulus to self-reflection and innovation, raising the level of performance across an enterprise. Do people get together on a semi-regular basis? This could take the form of formal grand rounds, conferences, seminars, and research colloquia. Equally important, however, are informal interactions around a water cooler or in a lunch room. Misinformed leaders may think we are reaping greater productivity by keeping colleagues so busy that such interactions cannot occur. In the short term, we are probably right. Longer term, however, we are eroding intellectual capital and undermining medicine's ability to respond creatively to future challenges and opportunities.

How often do people in our organizations see one another outside of work? People who have never had a conversation with one another are highly unlikely to form a collaborative relationship or develop a sense of shared community. Rising workloads and stress levels are threatening esprit de corps more than ever, and getting people together outside of work is crucial. Ideally, some of these interactions would involve not only department members but also spouses and children. It would be a healthy sign for a medical school or healthcare organization to find departments competing with one another to improve the quality of their intellectual community. When candidates come to interview, we should be showcasing our opportunities for intellectual growth and development. We should tout not only our equipment and facilities but also the liveliness of our intellectual interchange.

Physicians are intelligent people. We want to work in a place that provides real intellectual stimulation. Many of us are willing to trade income for an intellectually stimulating environment. We want to evaluate the quality of our work not only in terms of the number of patients we see, the amount of revenue we generate, or our number of errors, but also in terms of our level of intellectual engagement, and the extent to which we have been able to help identify both better ways of doing things and better things to do. One way of fostering such intellectual engagement is to get learners at all levels actively engaged in the life of the department. Are learners actively engaged in core departmental functions, such as residency recruitment and selection, budgeting, and strategic planning? Are they invited to participate in faculty meetings? Do they contribute to faculty hiring and promotion decisions? Treating learners as colleagues from the outset prepares them to make greater contributions when they assume formal leadership roles.

It goes deeper than this. To what degree are we turning to learners – medical students, residents, and fellows – to help us identify and solve the most pressing problems that confront our organizations? Are we inviting them to participate in identifying the most noteworthy opportunities before us? We make a great mistake if we confine learners' attention to studying books and passing examinations. They have real knowledge to share, and if we give them the chance, they learn from doing so. Our professional meeting programs and journals overflow with information about the latest scientific and technological innovations. Such novelties may at times eclipse everything else in our field of view. Do we even recognize new ideas about building intellectual community? How often do we pause to reflect on or to share our community-building approaches? If we fail to do so, medicine may be killing the goose that lays our golden eggs, and ceding the future of health care to other fields prepared to make such investments.

***

The great Danish philosopher Søren Kierkegaard (1813–1855), often considered the "father of existentialism," divided human life into three stages. He called these stages the aesthetic, the ethical, and the religious. At first glance such stages may seem rather far removed from the daily practice of medicine. Yet Kierkegaard's characterization of each stage helps to illuminate the challenges and opportunities before health professional today. By exploring each stage, we can clarify our vision of what it means to be a leader and help medicine to chart a more propitious course.

Kierkegaard (Fig. 9.2) was born and died in Copenhagen, Denmark. He studied theology at the University of Copenhagen,

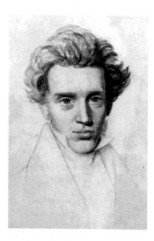

Fig. 9.2 Danish philosopher and theologian Søren Kierkegaard (1813–1855). Two of Kierkegaard's most notable lines are, "The tyrant dies and his rule is over; the martyr dies and his rule begins," and "You cannot get the truth by capturing it, only by its capturing you"

eventually earning a Ph.D. with a dissertation entitled, "On the Concept of Irony with Continual Reference to Socrates." One of the most notable features of his life was his relationship with Regine Olsen, a young woman to whom he proposed marriage yet soon thereafter broke off the engagement, citing his own tendency to melancholy. Kierkegaard's most widely read works are *Either/Or, Fear and Trembling*, and *Stages on Life's Way*. Before turning to Kierkegaard's account of life's stages, it is important to clarify one point. He did not regard these stages as mutually exclusive. In passing from the aesthetic stage to the ethical stage, or from the ethical stage to the religious stage, we do not completely abandon the preceding stage. Instead the aesthetic stage is incorporated into the ethical stage, much as a student might progress from arithmetic to geometry without forgetting how to add and subtract.

Kierkegaard's first stage is the aesthetic. The term "aesthetic" does not imply that people in this stage are all painters, poets, and musicians, although some certainly are. Instead the aesthetic individual is one who leads a life of sensation, characterized by enjoyment of passing interests and passions. One prototype of the aesthetic individual is the shopper, a person who takes great pleasure in visiting shopping malls or auto dealerships in pursuit of the latest style and technology. Another prototype of the aesthetic person is the gambler, who lives for the thrill of the wager. In the aesthetic stage, life amounts to a series of disconnected episodes. One night we go to the theatre, the next to the arena, and the next to the disco. We are moved by what we happen to enjoy, and the prospect of enjoyment is the thing that seems most real and worth living for. We are like people in an amusement park progressing from thrill ride to thrill ride. Beneath the excitement of the moment, however, we are inevitably plagued by an inner sense of ennui, from which each passing amusement provides only temporary distraction.

What is the relevance of the aesthetic stage to leaders? Anyone who has visited a large medical trade show can attest to its aesthetic dimensions. We roam from booth to booth, marveling at the latest devices and drugs, contemplating their use in our practice. Abetting us in this fascination is a healthcare system that strongly rewards the adoption of innovations, even if evidence concerning their efficacy and costs is limited. The aesthetic life is about calculation, not commitment. The goal is not to determine whether or not we really need the product, but how we can acquire as much of it as possible at the lowest possible price. As we move from vendor to vendor, we overlook an important truth, one readily accessible through a simple thought experiment: what if we had a bottomless budget? What if we could buy everything in the store? To what extent would our lives, and those of our patients, truly be enriched?

The aesthetic stage is inherently limited. The thing that interests us most at any particular moment is not necessarily the thing that we most need to attend to. According to Kierkegaard, a life devoted to such pursuits is a life suffused with world weariness, a weariness that leads eventually to despair. Whether our ambition is directed toward a journal article, a research grant, a teaching award, an office in a professional organization, or the most cutting-edge imaging technology, our acquisitions remain hollow unless they are situated in a deeper commitment. To appreciate the superficial nature of the aesthetic stage, Kierkegaard advises us to play the role of vendors ourselves. So long as we remain strictly on the purchaser end of such relationships, we will continue careening from acquisition to acquisition. Once on the vendor side, however, we can begin to see ourselves in the eager eyes of others. Only then can we experience the hollowness of such a treadmill life, running harder and harder but never really getting anywhere. Whatever genuine fulfillment means, it is not something that we can be sold, awarded, or elected to.

A deeper level of fulfillment opens up when we progress to the ethical stage. In this stage, our interest is no longer confined to the entertaining. Instead we feel a calling to know goodness and to seek genuine direction in life. We sense the need to commit to something, something whose worth exceeds our own. Some people encounter the distinction between the aesthetic and the ethical upon becoming a parent. A child provides a new locus of concern and commitment, in comparison to which life before children can seem both carefree and careless. Another example is marriage, which may lack the excitement of an unending series of new romantic adventures, but makes possible a far deeper and ultimately more fulfilling life. According to Kierkegaard, the challenge before us in the ethical stage of life is not to bend our will to some external set of policies, rules, or laws. Instead it is truly to become who we really are. Once we undertake this commitment, it becomes very important to lead lives that are consistent and coherent. Were we merely to flit from fad to fad, as in the aesthetic stage, we would be implicitly admitting that we have no self, no one we are meant to be. Underlying this argument is the assumption that we are not at liberty to decide who we are. There is someone that we are meant to be. The question is this: will we commit to becoming that person?

To live in the ethical stage is to live by ideals. What does it mean to be human, and what would a fully human person look like? What does it mean to be a physician, and what is our image of a truly great doctor? To suppose that a physician is a mere lesion detector would do medicine a great disservice. Such a physician would be a mere technician, operating at a purely technical level, the aesthetic stage. A physician is bound by the nature of the patient–physician relationship and the moral compact between medicine and society to pursue a higher ethical ideal. If Kierkegaard is correct, each of us harbors a deep awareness of the difference between making money and doing what is best for our patients and the community. Likewise, we know the difference between getting the work done and doing it to the best of our ability, as we hope a colleague would care for a friend or loved one. Here is the crucial question: will we devote ourselves to clarifying and realizing that vision in our daily practice?

In the ethical stage, we no longer seek to distract ourselves from the burden of self-assessment. Nor is our self-assessment confined to the question, "Am I having fun yet?" Instead we are committed to self-assessment in a deeply moral sense: Are we living up to who we really are? Everything we do flows from who we understand ourselves to be. Here Kierkegaard's role as a founder of existentialism comes clearly into view, for the call to live up to our ideal self is, in the final analysis, a call to live authentically.

Kierkegaard regards the religious stage as the highest level of human existence. He believes that it is possible to be ethical without being religious, but impossible to be religious without being ethical. To live in the religious stage, it is necessary to recognize human finitude, our inability fully to comprehend reality and our place in it. People who believe that human beings can completely understand the universe are unable to reach the religious stage, and in fact have no desire to do so. This transition is possible only for those who have plumbed the limits of human ken. Only having acknowledged that the highest truth is beyond our understanding can we grasp the necessity of faith.

In *Fear and Trembling*, Kierkegaard calls the person who exists in the aesthetic stage a "slave," the person who exists in the ethical stage a "knight of infinite resignation," and the person who exists in the religious stage a "knight of faith." He describes the knight of faith through a story about a man who is passionately in love with a princess but knows they will never be together. The aesthetic individual gives up and learns to love someone else. The ethical individual does not abandon his love, but resigns himself to the fact that it will not be realized in this world. The knight of faith, by contrast, lives with the expectation that he and his beloved will be together in this life.

Kierkegaard was wrestling with ultimate questions of human existence, not medical science, technology, or practice. Yet his perspective illuminates important issues before medicine. The forward march of technology seems inevitable. Calculations of cost, efficiency, and 24-hour availability are likely further to widen the gap between patients and health professionals. The ethical response is to long for a bygone era when referring patients and physicians really got to know one another, while acknowledging that such relationships are more difficult today. From the ethical point of view, medicine can respond to eroding professional relationships only with resignation. The religious response, by contrast, is to keep practicing medicine as though we can not only sustain but also actually strengthen patient–physician relationships and to look for ways to make it happen.

When, like the aesthetic individual, we give up on something that we believe in, we foreclose the possibility that it will ever come to pass. When, like the ethical individual, we cling to our ideals yet resign ourselves to the fact that we can never realize them, we render them extremely unlikely. When, like Kierkegaard's knight of faith, we keep hope alive, and live as though such ideals could be realized in this life, we leave the door open. We remain receptive to the possibility that even as technology and economics pull us in other directions, opportunities to cultivate and strengthen professional relationships will present themselves.

Kierkegaard's three stages of life represent a call to authenticity, a summons to resist the temptation to become so ensnared by the many little things that we forget about the few big ones. The pursuit of greater security, ease, compensation, awards, honors, and elected offices can be very seductive. Whole years and even decades can pass us by before we realize that, pursued for their own sake, they are ultimately hollow. Even the ethical life can leave us feeling empty, if we resign ourselves to the impossibility of realizing our ideals and making a difference. From Kierkegaard's vantage point, the highest and best life for a leader, as for any human being, is to live with our eyes on the timeless, a realm of significance that stretches far beyond today's fashions to encompass whole generations both long gone and not yet born. Set in this context, what is the deepest and most enduring significance of Leadership in Healthcare? What truth and goodness could we hope to realize each day? It is in living hopefully that we lead the most authentic lives.

Bibliography

Argyris C, Schön D. Organizational learning II: theory, method, and practice. Upper Saddle River, NJ: Prentice Hall, 1995.

Aristotle. Complete works. Princeton: Princeton University Press, 1971.

Beck AT. Prisoners of hate: the cognitive basis of anger, hostility, and violence. New York: Harper Collins, 1999.

Beckett S. Waiting for Godot. New York: Grove Press, 1954.

Berwick, D. A primer on leading the improvement of systems. BMJ 1996;312:619–22.

Coles R. The Erik Erikson reader New York, NY: Norton, 2001.

Davenport TH, Prusak L. Working knowledge: how organizations manage what they know. Cambridge, MA: Harvard University Press, 1998.

Deming WE. Out of the crisis. Cambridge, MA: MIT Press, 2000

Eco U. Narrative structure in Fleming. In del Buono E, Eco U (eds.). *The bond affair*. London: Macdonald, 1966.

Edmondson A. Learning from mistakes is easier said than done. J Appl Behav Sci. 2004;40:66–90.

Eliot TS. Complete poems and plays. New York: Harcourt, 1952.

Ellis A, Harper RA. A guide to rational living. Chatsworth, California: Wilshire Book Co., 1975.

Gardner H, Csikszentmihalyi M, Damon W. Good work: when excellence and ethics meet. New York: Basic Books, 2001.

Gibbon E. The history of the decline and fall of the Roman Empire. New York: Penguin, 2000.

Goleman D. Emotional intelligence: why it can matter more than IQ. New York: Bantam, 1995.

Grant M. History of Rome. Upper Saddle River, NJ: Prentice-Hall, 1978.

Harvard Business Review. Harvard Business Review on organizational learning. Boston: Harvard Business School, 2001.

Helmreich, Robert. On error management: lessons from aviation. BMJ 2000;320:781–85.

Herzberg F. "One more time: how do you motivate employees?" Harv Bus Rev. 2003;81:87–96.

Kierkegaard S. Kierkegaard's writings. Princeton: Princeton University Press, 1988.

Larson, L. Ending the culture of blame. Trustee 2000;53:6–10.

Ludmerer KM. Time to heal: American medical education from the turn of the century to the era of managed care. Oxford: Oxford University Press, 1999.

McClelland DC. Human motivation. Glenview, IL: Scott Foresman, 1985.

McGregor DT. The human side of enterprise. New York: McGraw-Hill, 1960.

Milstein, A. Out of sight out of mind: Why doesn't widespread clinical quality failure command our attention? Health Aff 2003;22:119–27.

Mintzberg H. The structuring of organizations. Englewood Cliffs, NJ: Prentice-Hall, 1979.

Plato. Collected dialogues. Princeton: Princeton University Press, 1961.

Poe EA. 18 best stories by Edgar Allan Poe. New York: Dell Publishing, 1981.

Polanyi M. The tacit dimension. New York: Anchor Books, 1967.

Revans R. The ABC of action learning. Melbourne, FL: Krieger Publishing Company, 1983.

Santayana G. Reason in common sense. Mineola, New York: Dover, 1980.

Senge PM. The fifth discipline: the art and practice of the learning organization. New York: Doubleday, 1990.

Smith L, Rao R. New ideas from the army (really). Fortune 1994;130:203–208.

Strayer DL, Power ME, Fagan WF, Pickett STA, Belnap J. A classification of ecological interfaces. BioScience 2003;53:723–29.

The New English Bible. Oxford and Cambridge: Oxford University Press and Cambridge University Press, 1961.

Tocqueville, A. Democracy in America. Chicago: University of Chicago Press, 2002.

Vroom VH, Jago AG. The new leadership: managing participation in organizations. Englewood Cliffs, NJ: Prentice-Hall, 1988.

Walker GE, Golde CM, Jones L, Bueschel AC, Hutchings P. The Formation of Scholars: Rethinking Doctoral Education for the Twenty-First Century. San Francisco: Jossey-Bass, 2008.

Wheatley W. Good-bye, command and control. Leader to Leader 1997;5:21–28.

Index